BE HAPPY OR GET THE F* OUT

A Bipolar Success Story — and Your Guide to Hope, Recovery, and Designing a Life You Love

Phylecia Kellar

Ballin and Bipolar, LLC

BE HAPPY OR GET THE F* OUT

A Bipolar Success Story—and Your Guide to Hope, Recovery, and Designing a Life You Love

PHYLECIA KELLAR

Disclaimer: The author makes no guarantees concerning the level of success you may experience by following the advice and strategies contained in this book, and you accept the risk that results will differ for each individual. The purpose of this book is to educate, entertain, and inspire.

For more information: visit ballinandbipolar.com

ISBN (paperback): 978-1-962280-27-3

ISBN (ebook): 978-1-962280-26-6

If you're talking to Jimmy Fallon through the TV and you think Oprah is dressed up as a nurse to conduct research on you at the hospital you're in, you may be having a manic episode.

Here's a Gift Before You Begin

Be sure to visit my website and download all the free shit!

ballinandbipolar.com/free-resources

To my parents—

If it weren't for you, I'd be in an endless cycle of manic and depressive episodes, homeless, or dead. I will never be able to repay you for catching me when I fell.

Table of Contents

Preface

A Poem on the Aftermath

What do you do when you think your life is a lie?
When you question your entire existence, you just want to say goodbye.
Life is going right, we loved what we did, we loved what we knew.
But what happens when you are lost and begin to think that none of that was true?
You find yourself in a deep, dark place.
You don't go out, you can no longer keep the pace.
Everything was a gray cloud, a mist.
I couldn't get out of it—it was difficult to even exist.
The friends I had, the family I knew . . .
They never wavered; they were the glue.
How do you come out of this, what do you do?
Life as I knew it before was over.
How do you reinvent a girl, all the things gone that drove her?
I tried to live, I tried to believe.

But what I couldn't get past were the powers that be.
I found myself lost and felt so alone.
Why me, why was I the one chosen? It seemed my life was indefinitely postponed.
When I couldn't laugh, smile, or comb my hair, my mother was there.
My mother saw me, she saw me completely bare.
I remember the day, the worst day of my life.
I suddenly arose and couldn't take all the strife.
Make it stop, make it stop, I said.
There was nothing anyone could do.
I had to get these terrifying thoughts out of my head.
When the dust finally settled, the clouds weren't as gray.
I tried to then come back and put those feelings at bay.
As the months went by, I could finally see that maybe, just maybe, there was some hope.
It took a lot of time, but I finally learned how to cope.
I began to see myself again, although things were quite different.
It would never be the same.
As the medication and therapy were working their course,
I would then be able to laugh without too much force.
A few years go by, and while this path was terrifying, lonely, and cold,
I was finally able to let go and begin to take hold.
Now, twelve years later, with some experience and wisdom,

I can go about my day, as myself, the Phylecia we all knew and loved,
I was finally able to march along to the beat of my own drum.
Never lose hope, as scary as it may get.
You are important, you are worth the fight.
Go on, grab your life by the horns and let in your own light.

Introduction

Life itself is hard enough. Can you imagine being bipolar at the same time? That's what bipolar people think, I'm sure, and I'm one of them. Life is hard enough for the mentally healthiest person on the planet. Can you imagine navigating life if you're not even stable? Can you imagine being fired, suffering loss, and going through breakups when your brain has a chemical imbalance? Can you imagine trying to cope when your brain tells you lies and turns off a function that helps you complete daily tasks? What about when mania tells you not to sleep or eat, and you have an energy level so high that it scares people?

This is my experience. I'm going to share with you how I got diagnosed with bipolar. I'm going to share the aftermath of a manic episode that I had in 2010. We are going to go through what happened after the diagnosis—what I call the fall, and my accompanying loss of identity. Then, I'm going to share my methodology to successfully overcome such episodes and live your best life.

I am ballin' with a little side of bipolar. Managed in a healthy way, being bipolar brings character to the day. That's what I want for you.

I am by no means a doctor. I am by no means a psychiatrist. I am an expert in this field because I fucking lived through it and am building my dream life as we speak.

I want other people to be able to learn from their bipolar disorder and accept it—but not in the sense of letting it lie. I mean I want you to understand your diagnosis, while also understanding there are *solutions.* There are solutions for depression; there are solutions for mania.

There are ways that we can be in love with being alive. That's one of my favorite things to say: I'm genuinely in love with being alive. I'm thankful for my diagnosis because it got me where I am today.

It also made me learn about myself and other people, and I now use that knowledge as a tool. I think bipolar people are creative. I believe bipolar people have a gift. But we have to use that gift in the right way.

We're going to explore the foundation of life itself, along with the component of being bipolar.

In January 2010, I was diagnosed with bipolar I. Unbeknownst to my family, parents, or friends, for eight days, I was in an acute mania to a delirious manic episode.

After an episode like this, depression is the natural progression (which none of my family or friends knew at the time, nor did I).

Your brain goes through severe trauma that it will take years to recover from (which, again, we didn't know at the time).

But what goes up *must* come down, and down I went.

What I needed back then was hope; I needed someone to tell me I had been through colossal trauma and that there was a way back.

But I didn't hear any of that.

I needed to talk with someone who had been diagnosed with bipolar I, someone who had been in my shoes and had come out the other side. I needed a bipolar success coach to save the day. That's why I'm here.

I didn't know it then, but my mission statement was born through these moments.

I wrote this book because in my hour of desperation and need, I called on a doctor, and he broke my heart. I needed hope, a plan, and a path. I had none. I was lost and heartbroken, and I felt alone.

You don't have to endure everything that I did. This book can be your yellow brick road, your hope, your plan, and your path.

I wrote this book for bipolar people everywhere. I wrote this book for people who struggle with mental health issues, anxiety, depression, and mania. I wrote this book for people who want to get better. You can learn about a fall from grace and the climb back up, knowing it's possible to adapt that approach to your own life. I wrote this book for family and friends of people who are bipolar.

You'll hear my experience firsthand, and you'll learn about tools, solutions, foundation building, and belief systems—but most of all, you'll have hope. You will not feel despair. You will know it's possible to come back stronger than your disorder ever was.

I also wrote this book because there are so many books by doctors who haven't walked in our shoes. I have. I have been you. My parents have been your family members.

I'm here to offer you concrete tools and solutions that will give you hope. By the end of this book, you'll know how to rebuild your life and what a true bipolar success road map looks like.

That's what we're going to do together in the following pages. It's your life; let's take ownership.

Let's go into every single day and fight for your life like Mike Tyson in the ring. You are worth every second.

A Friend's Perspective

Your diagnosis seems so long ago, and when I try thinking back on the events some of my memories are hazy, but at the same time I remember things like it was yesterday. I remember you had an apartment at that time. You've always had such an infectious and bubbly personality, so naturally everyone wanted to be there. One weekend night (I believe several days or one week before you were admitted), we had all been partying and drinking at your apartment and several people spent the night. I think we all stayed up pretty late before falling asleep, but I don't think you ever slept that night. I remember waking up early to leave the next morning, and you were still awake, hyperactively cleaning the kitchen and happily ranting about something. I forget exactly what you were talking about, but I remember your speech being rapid and frenzied—like you didn't have enough time to get everything out. I remember questioning to myself why you didn't seem drunk or even hungover.

Looking back, it's clear you were in a manic state. You were impulsive and had a lot of racing thoughts during that time. You were also going out almost every night, which never seemed to slow you down. You also had all of these ideas—some were delusional but nothing that would warrant concern—they were more like fantasies, dreams, and goals. You have always been optimistic and a dreamer at heart, so it wasn't too far off, but it was definitely on another level. I thought maybe it was normal—we were all young (nineteen to twenty years old) at the time and trying to figure out who we were and what we wanted in our lives. But still, something was off. I remember talking about you with someone (maybe Carolyn or Ian) and asking about things or if they seemed concerned—they too, had noticed the same behaviors.

Within a week, I got a call from your dad that you had been admitted to a psychiatric facility. They didn't know if you were suffering from bipolar or schizophrenia, but they were keeping you and starting you on medications. Your dad kept us updated, and I specifically remember him telling me that you had requested he bring you some new underwear since you were not allowed to leave. For some reason that always stuck with me. Maybe it was because at that time I finally realized the gravity of the situation, and that although you were an adult, you were unable to physically leave the facility. Your dad also said you seemed embarrassed when you asked him about the underwear—I never knew if he meant it was just because he had to go through your underwear drawer or if he was referring to your mental health and the stigma that is often accompanied with it.

When you were discharged, you returned home and lived with your parents. I remember visiting you pretty quickly afterwards, and we hung out in the living room just as we had in the past. This time felt different—you were there physically and looked well, but your entire personality was different. My once happy-go-lucky, hilarious, always-smiling friend was a shell of herself. You were subdued, barely smiled, and often stared off or at the ground. You had mentioned that they had been adjusting one of your medications (lithium?) and you didn't feel like yourself. It was clear you didn't really want to hang out or talk about anything. That night was difficult—I remember feeling helpless as I didn't know what to say or how I could support you.

The first year after your diagnosis seemed to be the hardest. They were still adjusting your medicines, so you still expressed "feeling off." The medication side effects also caused you to gain weight. You still weren't always open to having visitors or to hanging out. I had never seen you with such low confidence. Since I've known you, you have always radiated strength, confidence, and have been unapologetically yourself, so seeing you this way was hard and saddening. You didn't like to talk about your bipolar disorder or any of your emotions that were occurring at that time. There was nothing I could say or do to make you feel better.

I don't remember exactly when (maybe year two?), but it almost seemed like a switch was turned on and your demeanor slowly seemed to improve. You were becoming more social. You started telling jokes again, and your witty comebacks and silly expressions/sayings were back! I know they continued adjusting your medications, and it seemed like they finally got it figured out. You were smiling and truly seemed like you were happy. I think you got back into swimming and exercising at that time too, so it was awesome to see your confidence level return. I think you also started opening up about being bipolar, and it seemed like it was then that you finally accepted it and started moving forward with your life.

It's been over ten years now since your initial bipolar diagnosis. Looking from the outside, it seems like your bipolar has been well controlled. I don't know of any other manic or severe depression episodes that you may have had. You are still unapologetically yourself and as happy, caring, strong, confident, funny, and optimistic as ever. You're now open about your bipolar diagnosis and never ashamed to talk about it, which I think is respectable, amazing, and brave. You still have such an infectious and bubbly personality, and your support system proves that. I'm so proud of you and all of the work you have put into making yourself healthy. No matter what fight you may be facing, I will always be in your corner.

I love you, Phyl!
—Katie

Part I

The Manic Episode

Chapter 1
The Eight Crazy Nights

Let's go a little manic—whaddya say?

Let's go back to 2009 and 2010. I'm going to tell you the story as I remember it. You must know I suffered from blackouts, as my body couldn't keep up with my brain activity. If this seems choppy, that's because it was.

I had friends and other people around me all the time. I was super social and loved my life. I was in school full-time, served tables, had my apartment, and paid my bills. I worked hard and partied harder.

Around December 2009, I started talking in metaphorical terms. I still do that to this day. I love a good metaphor. It seemed natural.

I started saying things like "Oh my goodness, our lives are meant for something huge! We're meant for more!" It was almost like a switch went off. Then January came.

Slowly over the following weeks, people started to notice small things, but nobody could put their finger on it. Mania and what a manic episode looks like were not common knowledge among twenty-year-old kids in 2010. My situation was not a regular thing. The typical parent doesn't see their kid have a mental breakdown and say, "Huh, must be bipolar. Let's go get help."

(Note: Throughout this book, you'll read lots of football analogies—so get ready.)

Day 1: New Year's Day, 2010

(Note: There are stages to mania. In the first couple of days, I was in what's called "hypomania," or what I like to call the "peewee football" version of mania.)

I will pick up on New Year's Eve of 2009, going into 2010.

I was with Amanda and Anna, two of my closest friends at the time. Amanda, to her credit, saw a lot and would have done anything for me. I was a good ole pothead back then, but no other drugs were involved. We planned to go to Fourth Street Live, a big party place in our downtown with many bars. By this time, I had already lost a fair amount of weight. I wasn't eating much; it wasn't a priority. My priority was to smoke weed, talk, and party with friends. I didn't have much use for food. We had a great time that night!

The next part was strange, though. Don't get me wrong: I'd had my share of drunken blackouts. But this specific night, it was different. I was drinking and smoking some weed, but I did this regularly and had a good handle on what I could tolerate and what was too much.

I woke up the following day feeling different. I had lost hours. Something didn't feel right. It was different from a "drunken blackout." It was like space and time didn't make sense.

And I know what you're thinking: You were drunk and blacked out. But it wasn't that.

I knew that something was . . . off.

I learned later that when you're in a manic episode, you can suffer from blackouts or periods you don't recollect. This can be because your brain is running a thousand miles a second, and your body and memory simply cannot keep up. That's what it was for me—though we didn't know it then. After New Year's, I went about my day, but things got worse quickly.

Day 2: The Part Where I Quit My Job

My energy level was about to reach heights that would scare people.

This was like flying on a magic carpet ride with Aladdin and believing you're Jasmine.

On the second day, I quit my job at Cracker Barrel, which was a red flag. I never would have left my job on a whim without having another job lined up. I came into Cracker Barrel saying to all my server friends, "We're better than this! We are meant for more, y'all! I'm sorry, but I'm out." And I promptly left.

I started to believe that I was meant for "more," I had this notion that I was going to be famous. It seemed clear my first step in this venture was quitting my serving job, which was too low-level for where I was heading.

An awards show was happening that same day. I'm pretty sure it was the People's Choice Awards or the iHeart Radio Music Awards—one of those. I had invited about ten friends over. During this time, I was in a full-scale manic episode—but no one knew this.

I was frantically talking, and one of my friends later described it to me this way: "It's like you were trying to keep up with what your brain had going on inside, and your words couldn't keep up."

By this juncture, I believed that I would be famous, that I had arrived, and that all the celebrities knew about it. It was a world secret, but Phylecia was coming.

I kept saying, "We are going to be famous!" I remember people coming over and looking at me strangely. They began to leave with concerned faces.

These statements sort of sounded like me, but shit was getting weird.

I had always been energetic and loved the dream of "being famous," but my perspective was starting to become delusional.

I had friends over that night, and some of us were in my room. I had rapid speech. My brain was on fire, and sparks were flying off. My mouth was trying to verbalize what was happening in my head, but no one could keep up. I didn't have time to get all the words out.

In my world, I was trying to let people in on the news. Their friend Phylecia was going to be famous, and I had to tell them all about it.

My sister, Ashley, was the first to speak up. She stepped in and said, "Phylecia, no one knows what you're talking about; slow down. What is going on?"

I wasn't too keen on people questioning me. I went off. Now, my sister and I had fought in the past, but I wasn't one to just scream at her. I yelled at her to "get the hell out of my apartment" if she wasn't going to be on my level.

Ashley, who was only sixteen then, was scared and shaken. She called our mom, crying, and needed to be picked up.

My sweet friend Noelle listened and tried to follow what I was saying. You'll hear more about her later. She asked me if I could slow down and tell them what I meant or what I was trying to communicate.

I felt irritated and frustrated that no one seemed to understand me. "Why doesn't anyone GET THIS?!" I wondered. Why didn't they understand what I knew to be true?

In my world, the truth was obvious. If anyone questioned my state of mind, there was hell to pay.

Mariah Carey won an award that night. She talked to her fans during her speech and said, "I know who my true fans are."

I knew she was secretly talking to me—through the TV. She knew I was coming up and that I would be on her level soon.

Some people began to leave, and others stayed the night. I learned later that I didn't go to sleep that night. I never had a drink, and it didn't occur to me to smoke. I was too busy talking about my newfound celebrity status.

My friend said she woke up to me in the kitchen the following day, cleaning and talking to what seemed like myself. Still, she said nothing was slowing me down.

She spoke to our mutual friends, who agreed that something was off, but no one knew what. It wasn't quite time to call my parents. People were aware something was different, but again, who would think, "Hmm, it's probably bipolar, let's get her help"?

Day 3: Dr. Phyl

Let's hit on good ole Dr. Phil—or "The New Dr. Phyl," that is.

Back then, the TV therapist Dr. Phil was very popular. Well, my whole life, everyone has called me "Phyl." Also, my entire adult life, I had been a big player in my friends' lives, giving them advice and my two cents.

Anytime I walked into Cracker Barrel, there'd be five people at a time coming up to me, pumped to tell me about their days, their sexcapades, or the bitch at table 214.

"Phylecia! Oh, I need to talk to her. There's Phylecia. Hey, I need to tell you something!"

I took great pride in helping my friends, giving advice on their personal lives, listening, and laughing at everything everyone had to tell me.

This one night during my manic episode, somehow Dr. Phil came up. I had a revelation: *HOLY SHIT, that's it. I'm going to be the new "Dr. PHYL"! Get it? P-H-Y-L, Phyl.*

I got on my computer and emailed the Dr. Phil McGraw website team to let them know I was coming.

(I honestly don't know what I wrote them, but I bet it was wild, to say the least. What else could it have been?)

I had no credentials, but again, this was all a positively fantastic conspiracy that only I—along with Oprah, Dr. Phil, Jimmy Fallon, and Mariah Carey—knew about.

Oprah came in because Dr. Phil got his show thanks to her (or that was my understanding), so I had it all planned. If I wrote to Dr. Phil and said I would be on his show to "Dr. Phyl" it up, then Oprah would make me famous.

That was the beginning of the end. After that happened, we were on the fast track to being admitted to the damn mental hospital. Still, everyone was clueless as to what was happening.

Some people around me laughed and went along with it. My sister was in denial; if people asked her what was going on or came to her concerned, she didn't want to admit that anything was wrong with her big sister. *"Why can't you just be happy for her?"* she'd ask. *"She's just happy."*

She told me later that she began to question herself, wondering, "Does Phylecia really know something we don't?" No, I was just delusional.

Other friends were concerned but still couldn't put their finger on the problem. I didn't seem to be a danger to myself, and I wasn't hurting anyone . . . so what was the big deal? I'm sure some of them were thinking, "She's gotta calm down at some point, right?" Wrong-o.

Day 4: The Higher Power

(Note: We're now entering the world of college football—acute mania.)

Part of being in a manic episode is believing you are a godlike being. It's not so much that you *are* God as that you believe you are—or at least I believed that I was—some kind of angel or powerful spiritual being.

Here goes:

Remember, this shit didn't just come out of nowhere. Mania begins like a cute little seed in your head, because the thought is real to a certain extent. **Then it grows into about nineteen sunflowers in your mind, bursting with rays of yellow energy.** That's my definition of mania.

Let's go back to the fourth day.

I always had some number of people over. I had a couple of my close girlfriends and dudes with me. One guy I'd just met was in a deep conversation with me, or so I thought, and I was listening to his story. He was sitting in a chair, and I was sitting on the floor. I loved sitting on the floor—it kept me grounded (LOL, yeah right).

I began giving him some *wonderful* advice, or what I thought was wonderful. I remember thinking of him touching my hand as if to touch Jesus, and if he only touched my hand, he'd be a part of my light and sunshine.

Don't freak out; I didn't think I was Jesus, only *like* Jesus.

That doesn't make you feel any better, huh?

Let me try to explain. I was sitting there, and in my memory, the light was touching us, and it was a beautiful moment. And maybe it was! Maybe this dude and I were having a solid heart-to-heart.

This guy didn't know me; maybe he just thought that I was some crazy, funny girl who was

talking about all kinds of nonsense. It wasn't like everyone was terrified all the time; it didn't get like that until later.

These eight crazy nights progressed quickly, but at this point, I was life-of-the-party Phylecia—saying funny, off-the-cuff things, and full of way too much energy.

Note about this "energy": I didn't eat. I didn't sleep. *Eating and sleeping are unnecessary and a waste of time*, I thought. *I have too much going on for shit like sleep and food.*

The energy of mania is indescribable unless you've seen it. You cannot stop talking, you cannot sit down for any amount of time, you are thrilled, your thoughts are jumbled and racing all over the place—but the energy isn't stopping. Usually, the battery dies and there is a crash. (I came to find out there was a crash, but not until after I was forced to come down.)

This was an ongoing, undrainable battery on steroids that would soon have to be stopped.

Finally, back to Jesus. When he touched my hand (if he even did touch my hand—I could have imagined that one), I felt he was truly hearing what I was saying, taking it to heart. It felt as if the light shined on me, and in that moment, I felt like some kind of higher being.

I know this sounds weird, but it may sound worse than it was—or maybe it's exactly as bad as it sounds.

"You are welcome for my advice. Bless you, my child."

I'm kidding; I didn't say that.

Phylecia Kellar did not think she was Jesus. But I genuinely thought, *"Wow, is this what Jesus felt like when he helped people?"*

What was happening in my brain was very, very real.

Day 5: The Jimmy Fallon Conversation

We are on the fifth day of the eight crazy nights. Only three more days until the real shit hits the fan.

So, of course, I had people over, but as the night went on, they began to leave. Maybe a few people were over when this happened; I don't quite remember how many or who.

Jimmy Fallon, of course, had his late show. You know when the host speaks directly to the camera, and it looks like they're making eye contact with you?

Well, this specific night in January (and I don't know if Jimmy knows this or not), he was talking to me. That's right: through the TV, from New York City to Louisville, Kentucky, Jimmy Fallon himself knew that Phylecia Kellar had arrived. He knew that I was the up-and-coming star, and this was the best-kept secret since the Coca-Cola recipe. I knew I was going to be famous; he knew I was going to be famous. It was all starting to make sense now. He was part of the plan. I was going to be interviewed on his late show and couldn't WAIT.

As he spoke to me through the TV, I remember saying things like "*Yasss*, Jimmy, I know exactly who you're talking to. I will be there soon Jimmy, *YASSS*!"

As if I were responding *to* him. Now, don't get this confused with schizophrenia. All I'm pointing out is this is different. I wasn't hearing voices in my head; I was delusional. I believed things were happening that simply were not.

Remember, this was not drug-induced. I was too busy in my head thinking about how famous I was going to be to even worry about drinks or weed. I say this because the skeptics will say, "Ah, she was on drugs." And that's fine, but this was not the effect of hard drugs; this was a real-life attack of the brain, a short circuit in the wiring, my whole reality going off the rails.

I want to know what the neurons in my brain looked like. Could you see them going batshit crazy?

Day 6: The Sexual Encounter

On the sixth day of the eight crazy nights, I had one of my friends over, someone I had known for a while. He also worked with me at Cracker Barrel, so we had become close, everyday friends.

We had a relationship in which he would sometimes stay the night with me, but as I was a virgin at this time, there was no funny business, and he knew that. Everyone just knew "Phylecia doesn't do that."

My memory catches up around 2 or 3 a.m. that night. My friend was in my bed, asleep, while I was sitting on my couch, wide awake, writing frantically.

He woke up and noticed I wasn't in my bed. He walked to the living room and found me with papers everywhere, listening to Lil Wayne on my speaker system.

"Phylecia . . . What are you doing?" He said, concerned.

Why was I just sitting and writing frantically in my journal? Why was I so energetic and hadn't been to sleep yet? We both smoked weed together back then. He'd always be relaxed, and I'd get super energetic. That shit did not calm me down whatsoever. It only amplified my energy. I couldn't feel hunger, and I would laugh and love life. But in a manic state, it makes everything even more dramatic.

As we learned later, when your brain has a natural chemical imbalance, putting more chemicals on top of it? Not so great. Weed made the mania manifest faster and more aggressively (which I would come to be thankful for, a chapter for later).

I looked down at my journal, and it looked like I had a million thoughts; I had covered the paper, with words scribbled everywhere. There was no clear line of anything. It was just thoughts, quotes, and words in bold, scrawled all over the pages in big, crazy handwriting.

I remember saying, "Dude, I'm going to be a rapper like Lil Wayne." Back then, Lil Wayne was our *jam*. So I was going to be the peanut butter.

I had grown up Mormon (a story for later as well), so I was a virgin and still had it in my head that I didn't want to have drunken or meaningless sex with someone. Everyone knew the line I didn't cross. Having set the scene, here we go with the story.

I guess I finally "went to bed" and was *ready to go.*

When you are manic, things escalate quickly. You are not yourself. Rambling, euphoria, sexuality, and promiscuity come into play when they were never there before.

Mania is like being on a drug, but your brain is already chemically imbalanced, so ain't no drugs needed to feel like this.

I went back to my bedroom and hopped right on top of him—which I had never done in my life. You wouldn't have guessed it this night, though. You would have thought I was Samantha from *Sex and the City*, confident as hell and ready to pounce.

When I jumped on him, acting like someone completely different from the person he knew, even being a man, he had his reservations.

"Phylecia, are you sure? What's going on?" he asked.

My response: "Hell yeah, dude. Let's GO."

He was like "Alright, here goes."

To try not to be so graphic, let's just say that when the key was about to get into the lock, something came over me, and I hopped off and stopped.

People, I am telling you: that was an ABSOLUTE MIRACLE AND A GOD THING.

This was one of the most out-of-my-mind nights I had ever experienced, and somehow or other, my sane mind came to me and said, *"Phylecia, absolutely not. Get off this dude. You do not want to lose your virginity in this state, with this guy."*

To this day, it stuns me that I could come to and see what I was doing in my state of mind. I don't think it was me; I did not stop it. Somehow, something higher than me grabbed me and said, "This is not what you need to do." I paid attention.

I don't place blame on anyone here.

This part of the story is a textbook, poster-child manic episode. The only thing I think I *didn't* do was spend money. I never left my apartment because I had no real money to spend. However, I was told recently that I'd sent money to some nonprofit a few days earlier. I have no idea where.

I was just there in my own world, having the best time.

Day 7: Be Happy or Get the Fuck Out

Let me set this scene for you. On the seventh day, I was doing God-knows-what in my apartment all day. I'm sure I had people over at some point, maybe not. I know that I was blowing people up via text and phone calls this particular night. I posted all kinds of lyrics on Facebook.

My friend Nick commented, "Are you on drugs?"

My friend Jon said he woke up to eighty text messages. I must have had to tell him something vital.

My friend Amanda, one of my best friends at the time, worked the third shift at UPS. When she was at work, I never bothered her. I also never had her phone number at UPS; it was just her cell number.

If you knew me at all, you'd know that my door was always shut and locked. Not this time. It was the middle of the night, I had the music blaring, and my door was wide open.

I had called and texted Amanda all night at work. Somehow, I got the number to UPS and called her there.

When I did this, Amanda was instantly worried. She left work and came right over to check on me.

When she entered my apartment by way of the open door, she had a look of fear, worry, and concern.

I was a ray of golden sunshine and happy as shit. I did not want to be questioned.

She came in, and I saw the fear in her eyes. I still see those eyes to this day. They haunt me. I feel for her, knowing how she must have felt, what she must have seen. She lacked knowledge about what to do or what was happening with her friend.

She said, "Phylecia, I am so freaked out right now. What are you doing?! Your door was wide open? It's the middle of the night . . .? What is going on?!"

When she asked me this, I felt instantaneous anger. Mania can go from happy to pissed in a millisecond. Given the magnitude of the happy, endless energy, you can only imagine how it can escalate if someone is angry.

Yelling in the worst voice I have ever known, I responded to my scared friend:

"AMANDA, IF YOU'RE NOT GONNA BE HAPPY, YOU CAN GET THE FUCK OUT."

I proceeded to throw a cup at the wall.

Note: Amanda told me later, after everything was said and done that after I threw the cup at the wall, I hit her. I don't remember that, but don't know why she would ever lie.

Amanda left.

Day 8: Parents Find Out, Cops Are Called, and I'm Admitted to The Brook

(Note: Now we've entered delirious mania, or as I like to call it, the "Super Bowl" of a manic episode.)

Apparently, my close friend Jon had seen or talked to me, got worried, and tried to tell my sister that I needed help. She was in denial. He was the one who then got my dad's phone number and told him something was wrong and that I needed help.

Amanda was also part of this attempt to intervene; I think she called my mom.

My dad texted me, asking, "Are you on speed? Are you okay?"

I responded, "Yeah, dude! I'm just high on life! I don't need sleep." At the time, I guess I didn't.

Uncharted territory.

During this time, my dad worked in Lexington, about an hour away from where we lived. He called my mom after my friend called him. He told my mom to go check on me.

This was the first my mom had heard of this. She left her job at Walgreens, frantic and worried.

She knew I loved Taco Bell, so her strategy was to knock on my door with Taco Bell and act like she was just checking in with some food.

That didn't work, because I was not interested in food then. Recently, she told me that when she knocked on the door, she was worried right off the bat because, she said, "You were wearing a skimpy, tiny little tank top," which was not normal. It was crazy that I answered the door like that with no bra on. I was just out in my little skivvies, which was not me. She knew

I wouldn't have answered the door like that if I'd been in my right mind.

She looked around my apartment. It wasn't dirty, but there were journal pages, post-it notes, and other papers strewn everywhere.

She asked, "What's going on?"

Again, I was questioned and did not like to be questioned.

By the way, do you know those little metal scissors you can buy at Walgreens for eyebrows and nose hair? Well, I used to use those to shape my eyebrows. Pain is beauty, but not if you can help it. So, instead of plucking my eyebrows, I used those little scissors to cut them.

I had those scissors in my hand, and when my mom came to check on me, I said, "Mom, I have these scissors in my hand. I don't know what I'm going to do, but you need to leave."

She made a U-turn and left, setting the Taco Bell at my door. I remember that. From there, my mom was scared for me. She called my dad and didn't know what to do. She asked him, "What do I do?"

My dad said, "Well, I guess we call the police."

There was no book for dummies on a bipolar manic episode. No one knew what this was. *What's going on? Is she on drugs?* They knew I wasn't, but what could be happening? *Is she having a full-blown mental breakdown?*

Yes, that's exactly what happened.

Ultimately, we now know what it was, but at the time, they had no clue, and that's what the uncharted territory consisted of.

After this whole week of talking to the TV, thinking I would be famous, scaring people with my energy, blah blah—you now know the story—my dad said, "We need to call the cops, but I'm on my way there. Do not let them enter her apartment until I am down in the parking lot and until there's a female police officer with the other officer." He's smart enough to know that while I love a good police officer and I support the men in blue, there was a component of this situation that was scary. God only knew what mental state I was in and what it could escalate to. He would feel more comfortable if there was a female with the male cop, and he was right.

And by the way, we need a system with a mental health advisor to respond to calls like these, because the officers are automatically going to be on the defensive. Am I a danger to them, myself, or others? That's their job, and that's fine, but there are certain ways to handle mental health assessments and calls like these. But I digress.

My dad knew he wanted to be there. The cops came to my door. And somehow or other, I knew I needed to go with them. I knew that this was what was happening. I never questioned it. It was weird, because the scene could have gone very differently. I could have gotten defensive; I could have gotten violent. I could have gotten pissed, as I did with my sister or Amanda. But I think it was a God thing or a universe or whatever-you-believe-in thing.

In any case, it was odd because it was almost like in the state I was in, I knew I was going with the cops because this was part of the story. This was part of my becoming famous or whatever was happening in my brain. I thought that this was just part of that path. *I need to go with them because we're going to have a parade; they need to take me wherever I have to go.*

You must understand, I had *zero* grasp on the situation. I had no idea my friends were scared and had called my parents. I had no idea my parents were so freaked out that they had just called the police and filed a mental inquest warrant.

I was in my own little world, high on life and thinking I would be famous. I loved my life, and to me, this interaction with the cops was just part of the story.

So I got in the police car. They ended up driving me to the University of Louisville Hospital because they wanted to make sure that we could do the necessary blood work, urinalysis, and other assessments, I guess to confirm I wasn't on drugs. Unbeknownst to me, my parents followed the officers to the hospital; I had no idea they were anywhere to be found. The officers told my parents that in the car, I was talking away as if I had a friend back there, but I was by myself. They said, "She did not shut up the whole time. She was having an entire conversation. We don't know who she's talking to."

Really, I was just talking to them about how famous I was going to be, and I remember asking them to turn up the Fergie song that came on the radio: "Yo, can you turn this up?" Chapstick was a big deal, so I asked them if they had any Chapstick. I always need Chapstick to this day. And that's what it was in the cop car. I was just talking away, and they thought I was talking to myself. God only knows what those poor cops heard.

Then we got to the hospital, and again, I had no sense of the gravity or what this would all mean later—that this whole episode would derail my life in about a month. I was just in my own little world thinking I was going to be famous, not knowing it was a manic episode.

Before I end this chapter, let's close out the story.

I got to the hospital, and this was the wild part: I was in what looked like a closed-off waiting room with chairs, but there was nobody in it. I could see the nurse through a little window; I believed 1,000 percent that he was Dr. Phil's son. In my mind, it made sense he was researching me, because I was going to be the next Dr. Phil.

So okay, got it. So I'm here. They're going to research me so that they can interview me later. It's Dr. Phil's son. He's doing his research; it makes sense.

There was an African American lady who had Oprah's height and build, but she was wearing nursing attire. And I was like, *Oh my God, Oprah is here. Oprah is doing her research on me. This makes sense now.*

That's the state my brain was in. I was in this room, thinking, *Okay, cool. We got it all lined up. This is why I came. Oprah's back there doing her research. Dr. Phil's son is here. They're going to band together. We're going to do this whole episode and this interview, and then that's the launch of my famous career.*

The only time I got irritated was when nobody would tell me what the fuck was going on. So I kept asking, but who knows what types of questions I was asking? I wasn't asking normal questions. I was probably literally like, "Yo, where's your dad? I know you're Dr. Phil's son, so where's your dad at? Is he coming?" So, you have to put yourself in the staff's position too, because *who knows* the people, they see every single day on drugs or dealing with mental health issues? They just ignore those people, and I was one of those people that day. I got pissed because nobody would tell me what was going on, and I was in this room for a long time. I got physically uncomfortable and tried to sneak out to the beds down the hall, but the nurses kept telling me to go back to this little room. I was like, "Hello, those chairs are uncomfortable!" Then I would proceed right back down the hallway like a sneaky undercover boss. I just wanted to lie down. What the hell was going on?

I remember banging on the walls because I thought my friends and family were waiting for me for this parade we were going to have. "Hello! I'm in here. I'm in here!"

It's sad to think about, because bless my heart.

Later, this other lady was in the waiting room with me. She didn't have nice clothes on. She was missing teeth. She looked like she was having some trouble in her life, and she was in the hospital with me. You know, same story. So, who knows what was going on with her. She was thin, she was African American, and she was a woman. You'll see why I'm saying this in a second. In my mind, that woman in the waiting room with me was . . . wait for it . . . Michael Jackson.

Michael Jackson had died the year before, in 2009, which I was very aware of. This was 2010. I believed this woman was

Michael Jackson reincarnated. Yes, in reality, he was dead, and this was just a woman going through some struggles. But you must understand the brain I was working with then. I believed his spirit had returned somehow. I didn't think she had his body, but at the same time, I kind of did, because she was skinny like Michael Jackson. So, I believed she embodied his spirit. I kept telling her, "I know who you are, I know who you are," and pointing at her as if to say, "Props to you, I get you."

She said, "I'm whoever you want me to be, baby!"

And I was like, "Yeah, I know who you are."

Finally, after they had the results of my bloodwork and my pee test, I'm guessing they said, "Okay, she's not on drugs. She needs to go to the mental facility." I got in an ambulance to go to the mental health hospital in town.

Well, the last part of this whole shebang was when I was in the ambulance. I wanted Chapstick. Remember, Phylecia loves some Chapstick. The sweet lady in there with me was communicating with me. She was kind and empathetic to my needs. My grandma had died a couple of years before this, and I believed this person embodied my dead grandmother's spirit and was helping her little granddaughter get the Vaseline she needed for her lips in the ambulance on the way to the hospital. And maybe that's true. Maybe she did, and maybe my grandma was there in spirit. But I believed the emergency responder was her. I kept telling that lady, "Oh my gosh, I know who you are." The lady smiled and went about her business, being kind and chatting with me. To this day, I am so grateful for that lady, whether she was my grandma or not. She made me feel safe and was kind.

After that, my memory goes dark and blank. I don't remember going into the hospital. I don't remember taking medicine. I don't remember anything. They could have shot me up with something. I have no idea. In writing this, I want to call the hospital and ask. Did they give me a shot to come down? What did they give me? How much? What did I take? I just knew it was an ambulance, and then I came to The Brook and couldn't stand up. Say what you want, but I needed to come down somehow at the time, and that's what they did. I remember leaning against the wall. I couldn't walk or see; everything was a literal and figurative blur. It was like being on drugs. I mean, I was. They put me down. I was standing next to the wall and couldn't see straight or open my eyes. On the wall, and here we are.

Now, it's time for the aftermath. But to summarize what this episode meant, my entire life and being were about to change. I had no idea what was to come.

Takeaways

Mania is not just happy and energetic—it's scary. It can become dangerous. The only drugs I did back then were THC and alcohol, so for the skeptics, this episode did not result from using acid, coke, or speed. My brain took flight. But what goes up, must come down.

Chapter 2
Ten Days in a Psychiatric Facility

I Flew over the Cuckoo's Nest

So, I found myself in a mental hospital. They assigned me a psychiatrist. While I might have been on medications and might not have had the same energy as before, I was still very much in a manic state. My psychiatrist's name was Dr. Spears.

As I was talking to him, I thought he was Britney Spears's dad. So I said, "Oh, I know who you are. How's Britney doing?"

I'm sure he got a quick clue as to what was going on. My energy level wasn't wildly high, but I was still very much in a delirious manic state. I still didn't grasp the situation's gravity. I had no idea where I was. I just knew I was someplace, and I was talking to Britney's dad. *It's all part of the plan.*

We had meetings, and I still had no idea what was happening. I remember being in a room with people talking about my life.

We left the second-floor ward and went down to the cafeteria to get lunch. I was sitting there thinking, "Oh, there's a door. I can just walk out this door."

In truth, I'd been signed in, and I could not leave. I tried to walk out the door, and the alarms went off. They put a red band on me and sent me back upstairs. I couldn't come down to get food for a day because they thought I would try to escape! I wasn't trying to escape. I just saw a door and thought I could go home. For twenty-four hours, I was on a hold, so my meals were brought up to me. I thought it was cool, because I like meals brought to me. To-go food is my shit.

As I was writing this, my mom said, "Do you remember calling me?"

I said, "Not really." I knew I made calls when I was there, but I don't remember the details.

I remember getting out of the hospital and telling my friend Allie, "I'm sorry I didn't call you while I was there."

She said, "Phylecia, you did call me, multiple times. We had conversations. Do you not remember that?" Blackouts and short-term memory loss are what apparently happens in these episodes.

I'd called one of my guy friends to come get me. I was like, "Yo, man! I'm good. Just come pick me up!" He tried—and failed. Swing and a miss. He called my friend Jon, who told him, "Dude, you can't pick her up. She's legit admitted."

That was a hard truth and reality that even my friends couldn't fathom.

I called my parents when I arrived, not really knowing why I was there. I didn't know what being admitted meant. I had no idea what bipolar was. That word had not even been spoken at that point. I had a whole ten days left to go in the facility.

On the first or second day, I called my mom and said, "Hey! I'm ready to come home now! You can come get me."

She said it was sad because she didn't know what to say. She could tell I obviously didn't know why I was there. She told me, "You had no idea that we had to call the cops on you and that we filed a mental inquest warrant. You had no idea what was going on."

My mom didn't know what to say. She replied, "Phylecia, you can't come home yet, honey. You have to stay there for a little bit." My mom said she felt really sad about that.

Another piece of this is I wanted to talk to my sister on the phone, but she was so scared. She was freaked out about the whole situation. I said, "Hey, is Ashley there?" Later, I found out my sister didn't want to talk to me. Not out of anger—she was out of her depth. The idea of talking to me made her anxious. I think she was questioning a lot. But she knew that her sister was not okay.

For her whole life, I'd been her older sister who had it together. When I got admitted, it was scary for her. If she had talked to me, I probably would have told her some off-the-wall shit and said, "Hey, come get me." She didn't know what to say, so she opted out. She did not talk to me for about a week. I think she came to the hospital and visited me, but it was a little bit later.

I remember having a good time at the mental hospital. I describe my experience there by saying they were trying to get my brain to calm down. My brain was on fire when I arrived. For the first couple of days, I was still very much in a manic state and unaware of what was going on. It takes a long time for brain activity to slow down.

I was working with a psychiatrist. The first step was getting diagnosed. My diagnosis ended up being bipolar I. I'd just had a manic episode, and now the goal was to try different medications to level my moods back out. There would end up being a long road ahead, years of correction and leveling out. But we were still in the initial phase.

My dad told me they were trying to calm me down and had given me so much medication, but it was not working. They gave me at least three times the amount that other people are given in a manic state like this, yet I was nowhere near calm. "She's still the same," they would tell him after two more rounds of meds. You can only imagine what kind of horse tranquilizer they had to freaking give me to calm my ass down.

I could no longer fall asleep on my own. Falling asleep naturally was now a distant memory, a thing of the past. I needed meds to turn off my brain.

I want to make something clear: this was all very new. I was watching the show *Nurse Jackie*, and in that show, Nurse Jackie goes to rehab. She was an addict and wanted to get out of rehab early. She told the woman who ran the facility that she had thick skin and could handle it.

The woman said something to the effect of: "Not now, you don't. You used to. When you walk outside, the air will hurt your skin and you won't be able to breathe."

Once you're admitted, you don't have thick skin anymore. And rehab is an incubator. You are given everything. It's a confined space. It's a controlled environment where you have a schedule and a therapist right at your fingertips. All of this was relatable to my time at The Brook. You have people waking you up for breakfast—*and then we're gonna go color, and then we're gonna have group therapy, then we're gonna have one-on-one therapy.* You're not living your real life. This is not the real world. It's only meant to calm us down enough to function in real life. That's all it is: a pause in reality. Then you're supposed to go back to life as you had known it before.

Ultimately, The Brook was rehab for my brain. I went through some heavy trauma. I wasn't aware of the fact that I'd been diagnosed with a disorder. I wasn't aware that I would be on medication for the rest of my life because my brain has a chemical imbalance. I wasn't aware that my life would be different.

When I got out of The Brook, I had no idea what was to come—but that thought wasn't even alive yet.

I had just spent ten days in a mental hospital, and I was now on three very strong medications. I had no idea how hard it would be to just live, to be me again.

The only thing I knew the moment I was released from the hospital was that something had happened; I just wasn't quite sure what. I needed to be in that place for a couple weeks, but all in all, I felt pretty good! I was ready to go home.

I was never even told I was bipolar, or if I was, it was a fleeting comment that didn't sink in. I wasn't told what had happened. I should have stayed at the facility for much, much longer, until I understood fully what had happened, but this place was expensive.

They had me stay ten days to come down from that magic carpet ride, but it would be up to me to navigate the rest.

I had no idea depression was coming or how hard it would be to overcome. I had no idea just how much the aftermath of this episode was going to affect my life. I had no idea that I would one day be crying so hard and be scared for my mom to leave for work because I needed her with me all the time. I had no idea that I would begin to question my life and who I was. I had no idea that my sister and I wouldn't speak for a year.

I had no idea walking out of The Brook that times when I'd been smiling and laughing would feel like distant memories of another person.

I had no idea how hard it would be to take a walk, to shower, and to maintain personal hygiene.

I had no idea how hard it would be to talk, to laugh, and to put on a happy face for friends in hopes that they wouldn't see how unbelievably sad I was.

I had no idea how hard it would become to communicate or to remember fun times without wanting to cry, to remember who I used to be and to know I was no longer that person.

Takeaways

I want you to understand that my struggle was Stage 1 of the Bipolar Life Cycle (more on this in the next chapter). Flailing could be mania, hypomania, or a full-fledged manic episode that can derail your life.

I was flailing. I had no idea what had happened, nor did anyone around me. I was lucky enough to have good friends and amazing parents.

Even though I may not have been wildly energetic and delirious, I still did not understand the gravity of the situation I had found myself in. I was clueless. I thought that I was going to go back to life as I had known it, and I just needed to be on some meds now.

I was sorely mistaken.

I will leave you with this: people are not just crazy. Don't dismiss them as being crazy.

Mental illness is real, and I will not shy away from it. Far too many people do, and far too many people suffer for this not to be talked about. If I must shout these stories from the rooftops in order to get through and help one person with this disorder, I will.

I want people to know what I went through—it was real. It was raw and wild. It was sad and heartbreaking. But I came out of it, and you can too. You never know what tomorrow may bring; it may be perfect, or it may be terrible.

Put your game face on.

Chapter 3

Here's What Just Happened

The Stages, Cycles, and Seasons of Getting Diagnosed Bipolar

Allow me to introduce you to what I call the "Bipolar Life Cycle." For the rest of this book, I'll consecutively cover every single stage and my experience with each one, including the pivotal moments that changed mindsets, where I was searching, where I was flailing and lost myself, and how I climbed out of it inch by inch, day by day.

Your experiences will be a bit different, but the overall cycle is the same. I want you to get your journal or notebook out, write down what each stage means to you, and examine your experience. This will help you understand your own triggers and solutions, allowing you to build your own foundation. When I first got diagnosed, I was desperate for someone to give me hope, but no one did—or no one *could*. I'm here to give you the road map I longed for.

Here's to you and fighting for your life.

The Bipolar Life Cycle

(Note: This can be downloaded and made your own, along with other freebies, at ballinandbipolar.com/free-resources.)

Your cycle and pivotal moments will be individual to you, but they'll still have similarities to my experience, as the basis is the same. Pivotal moments can be as simple as knowing you have a problem that needs fixing or as significant as shifting your whole mindset.

Here we go.

1. **Flailing:** You ask yourself, *What just happened?* This could be hypomania, acute mania, delirious mania, or what is known as a manic episode.

2. **Aftermath:** This stage includes depression, pity ("Why me?"), blame, sadness, anger, and guilt. Reality hits.

3. **Acceptance and Surrender:** Stability is your number one job. You're in survival mode. This stage is about finding routine, adjusting meds, working with a psychiatrist and therapist, assembling your dream team, mapping out your plan, and being intentional about how you approach each day to fight for your life. It's important to pay attention to

your physical health, through exercise, eating right, sleep, and hygiene. These are basics that we must nail; they must become second nature. I know this sounds like a lot right now but remember: *baby steps.* One day at a time.

4. **Learning How to Breathe Again:** This stage is about managing your diagnosis the right way, finding solutions for mania and depression, understanding your triggers, knowing how you feel when mania is beginning, and understanding what depression is. What are you going to do when mania or depression hits? You must know what calms you down, what brings you up, and what your coping skills are. At this point, we are taking responsibility for our lives—and taking control. Take ownership, because no one is coming to save you but yourself. There's a mindset shift from pitying yourself and asking, "Why me?" to empowering yourself and asking, "Why not me?"

5. **Climbing Back Up:** Here's where you build or repair and then begin to rely on your foundation. This stage is about finding confidence, independence, and joy. You have to know where you want more confidence, how you can feel independent, and where your joy is. In your first go-round with this stage, you might just be happy as hell that you were able to fill up your gas tank

with your own money. Later, you might be pumped that you got a promotion. We get more advanced as we continue to progress.

6. **Learning Who You Are:** This stage involves searching, clarifying your belief system, and identifying your morals. What do you stand for? What do you *not* stand for? What are you going to put up with in life? Are you going to stand for something—or fall for anything?

7. **Gratitude:** Looking back on where you've been and how far you've come, you can be thankful for the good days or even the mediocre days in a way that you took for granted before. It's time to find gratitude and joy in the small things. Celebrate that you've gotten through some hard shit.

8. **Learning How to Be in Love with Being Alive:** Remember to laugh every day. Engage in professional development. Build real relationships and get rid of toxic people. Do the next right thing. Once we're not just surviving, we can ask who we want to be for the rest of our lives. What do you want to bring to the table that is life? Once you are stable and have a plan, life can flourish. What does this look like for you? Practice conflict resolution—the only way you can control anything is through how you react. How can

you see a difficult situation differently? Perspective is everything. Get your priorities in place and rely on your values. Stay focused on your vision for the future.

9. **Thriving:** By this stage, we have plan and a road map. We know our triggers, where we want to go, and what we want to improve on. It's time to take leaps! As Rachel Hollis says, do something that makes you say, "Holy shit, *I* just did that." Do something you've always wanted to do but previously told yourself you couldn't. As long as it's safe, happy, and healthy, *rock on*. Engage in continued education. Challenge yourself, but always work on staying centered. We cannot forget that we're bipolar. We will flail again, and we will feel depressed again—but now we have the tools to get out of it in hours rather than days, weeks, or months.

   Your mental health and taking care of your brain and body are part of the daily game. You know what you're going to do, while also working toward your bigger dreams beyond bipolar. Just because we're bipolar doesn't mean we can't be ballin' like anyone else. Any time you flail or become depressed, go right back to basics and start the cycle again. You'll soon get through it quicker and quicker. The clouds won't be so dark, the dark episodes won't be so long, and soon, they may only come every few years.

Live your life like you're singing your favorite song alone in your car on the best day. As the saying goes, "Dance as if no one is watching. Sing as if no one is listening." Be your own main character.

10. **Pivotal Moments:** That mindset alone is everything. When you believe in yourself and start to try more, you can do more than you ever thought possible.

    Pay attention to your own pivotal moments. These moments and mindset shifts for me have been life-changing. Go back through your life and see where those moments were. For me, the first moment was when a switch flipped. After years of feeling bad for myself, feeling guilty, and blaming the world, I stopped asking, "Why did this happen to me?" I accepted my path and started finding purpose in it. *Lightbulb.*

As you move through these stages and climb out of survival mode, thriving and falling in love with being alive represent the ultimate goal. You find your footing and learn more about yourself, until bipolar becomes just a part of you, without defining you.

Then you're untouchable.

What Even Is Bipolar?

Bipolar is sort of like diabetes, in that there is a type I and a type II.

Type I

Bipolar I is defined as having a week-long manic episode at least once in your life, or manic symptoms that are so severe you need immediate medical care. The mania involves an extreme change in mood and cognition that can interfere with school, work, or home life. The mania is then followed by terrible bouts of depression, which typically last for at least two weeks.

Phylecia's Definition: Bipolar I is a week-long manic episode that derailed my entire life, and I had to rebuild everything from scratch.

I want to touch on the stages of mania. If you remember the manic episode, I described in chapter 1, these stages happened to me exactly.

From December into early January, I was experiencing what's called *hypomania.* Hypomania could be defined as a normal person having the best day, with high energy, happiness, and rapid speech (peewee football).

Then I evolved into *acute* mania. In this phase, we are very unstable. This is where I began to believe I was going to be famous and when I started responding to Jimmy Fallon through the TV, as if he were talking to me directly. Acute mania is described as extreme instability and euphoria, along with irritability, reckless behavior, promiscuity, excessive energy, and highly rapid speech (college football).

Then we enter the world of *delirious* mania. This is where I was by the time I got to the hospital: totally out of touch with reality. This stage is defined as being in an altered state of consciousness (the Super Bowl). In my case, I believed that a parade was happening, that my dead grandmother had been embodied by my nurse, and that Michael Jackson, who had died the year prior, was a homeless lady in the room with me—if that's not delirium, I don't know what is.

So this puts mania in perspective. It's a progression.

Side effects and signs of a manic episode can include:

- feeling very happy, elated or overjoyed (I'll add: and if others around you aren't happy, they can get the F* out.)
- using rapid speech (speech so fast that no one can understand or keep up)

- feeling full of energy (like sunflowers bursting with sunshine in your brain and being led by the Energizer Bunny who never tires and needs no sleep or food)
- feeling self-important (godlike)
- feeling full of great new ideas and having important plans (I was going to be famous—I just knew it.)
- being easily distracted
- being easily irritated or agitated (to the point where people become fearful and very worried)
- being delusional, hallucinating, and experiencing disturbed or illogical thinking (delusions of grandeur that make no sense whatsoever)
- spending excessive money
- engaging in uncharacteristic promiscuity

I was the poster child for a manic episode, but no one knew it at the time. It makes sense that I'd be bipolar, as I had naturally high energy and always knew I wanted to do something big. The mania came on naturally but got progressively worse.

Type II

Bipolar II is not as severe or "dramatic" as bipolar I. It is defined by having highs and lows, and suffering from the hypomania described above—a more mild form of mania, usually elevated energy and hyperactivity. You don't go through a full-blown, severe manic episode. The mania affects thoughts, mood, and behaviors and may not last as long as episodes in bipolar I.

While it seems good that bipolar II is not as dramatic, it's harder to diagnose. It can also be misdiagnosed, for instances as just depression or as ADHD. It's harder to know what's going on.

By contrast, bipolar I is very easy to diagnose because it is so prevalent and obvious (to doctors). However, it is harder to treat, as it takes time to come down. When you do come down, it can take days, weeks, months, or years to regain control.

Usually when people are diagnosed bipolar, they are given medication to get level. Medication is no cure-all, but it can help to make the mania and depression less dramatic. It is there to help you get stable, though you must still work internally, physically, and emotionally as well to make a full recovery.

From the book *BIPOLAR, Not So Much* by Chris Aiken MD. and James Phelps, I learned important information that you should know about depression. In the book, they mention that "there is something in your brain that triggers behaviors to keep you on task and help you function as a human. That part—the limbic center—tells us to take a shower, to go to work, to take care of our kids. The brain passes information from the thinking center frontal lobes to this emotional center."

The authors continue, "This process allows people to move easily through their days, making good decisions, staying on task, and keeping up with daily priorities. In a healthy brain, this engine runs the show. During depression, though, the engine is turned off. As a result, everyday tasks seem impossible, and simple decisions seem paralyzing."

Depression also lies. It will tell you that you are a piece of shit, that you can't live a normal life, that you can't do the laundry today, and that you just need to stay in bed. In all actuality, you *can* do these things, but you're in a battle against your own mind.

You cannot think your way out of depression. Your brain got you there in the first place, so you cannot depend on your brain alone to get you out.

You must now find solutions to distract from this mindset and come back in a positive way.

Takeaways

Mania is wild. There is a progression to a manic episode if you have bipolar I.

The more you understand the disorder itself, the better the recovery becomes in regaining control of your life.

Depression will lie to you. You can make a comeback.

Chapter 4
Who I Was Before

Before Manic Episode

To give you a little bit of background on me, I grew up very social. I never had anxiety or depression—or even knew what those words meant.

I was on a United States swim team in high school and always had a lot of friends. I was always happy. I never struggled with my emotions. I freakin' loved my life.

I had a great time in high school and growing up. I moved to Utah when I was eighteen; I grew up Mormon, and that's what you do apparently.

The life I knew was easy-peasy lemon-squeezy. I had a great family, including my sister, who is four years younger than I am. I loved to make people laugh and make others feel good.

By 2009, I was living back in Kentucky, sharing an apartment with a friend. I was in school full-time, served tables, and partied full time. I was independent, paid my own bills, and was living my best life. Or so I thought.

I'm setting the scene for you here, so you'll see the full picture of my life before shit went down. We always had people over to our apartment. We were servers, and people would always come over after work. We'd laugh and talk for hours. It was a very social environment.

I went to school on Tuesdays and Thursdays, so I would work Monday, Wednesday, Friday, Saturday, and maybe some Sundays for the breakfast crowd. We would work doubles and make rent in a weekend. We were young, and we were living the fast life. It was so much fun.

I drank back then, but weed was everyone's BFF. We would smoke and go into work high as hell, asking each other, "Do I look high?"

"Yeah, you look high," someone would say. "Ya smell high, and your eyes are red as shit." But we rocked on and killed it every day. We worked hard and played harder.

We didn't do hard drugs. There was no Adderall or cocaine around. It was THC and alcohol—that's it.

Before my episode, I could go into work and have ten people talking to me. I could listen to every single person and respond with eagerness. I never got overwhelmed. I never got nervous about much. I got stressed out like any person as a server or with school tests, but that's about it.

I constantly had people over to my apartment, but I was also happy to be alone. I was comfortable in my own skin and loved who I was. I always had a sense of confidence and a positive, upbeat vibe around me. I was attracted to people who had big personalities and who loved to dance, laugh, and hang out—and those kinds of people were attracted to me.

One of my favorite things to do was drive around with my friends, listening to music and smoking Black & Mild cigars. We had a great time. We loved listening to comedians like Katt Williams and Dane Cook.

I loved my parents and was open with them about my life. I knew who I was, and I loved who I was. I was Phylecia.

Takeaways

You need to know a quick synopsis of who I was before so that you can fully understand what happened after. I was not on hard drugs. I was social and had many friends, whom I spent time with daily. I was happy and loved my life.

What happened after my manic episode is something I would never wish on my worst enemy.

Part II
The Aftermath

Chapter 5
Life as I Had Known It for Twenty-One Years Was Over

(I Just Didn't Know It Yet)

Life as I'd known it two weeks prior had ended.

That doesn't mean it was a death sentence. But it means that, number one, the reality that I had known for twenty-one years of my life was over. It is a hard reality and a harsh truth to come to understand that you have a disorder in the first place. Number two, I'd have to be on medication for the rest of my life to function normally.

When you get this diagnosis, now you must focus on your mental health and being stable, along with all the other shit that life throws at you.

I was at the facility for ten days. I still had no real grasp of the situation. I went through the motions, had fun, and made friends. I had a little goodbye party. When I got home, it still took a few weeks for reality to set in, for me to even realize what had happened and what it all meant. When I got home, I was still thinking about this parade. I knew that it was probably not real, but the thought was still there.

When I got home, I was thinking, *I'm just gonna go back to life as I knew it. I'm gonna go back to work. I'm going to live life like I always have.*

I was sorely mistaken.

The truth hit me like a ton of bricks, because no one told me what would happen. No one told me what was normal. That's why I do what I do now: because people need a path. You need to see the light at the end of the tunnel. Not only did I have no idea what was going to happen, I had no path forward. That is the gap I want to acknowledge. When I got out of the hospital, I thought that I was gonna go back to life as I knew it—if I just took some medication, everything was going to be fine.

That was not the case.

As the weeks went on, I knew that I had to take pills now, including a certain one to fall asleep. That's about it.

Things started going off the rails when I went back to work. I got my job back at Cracker Barrel, but I could not handle it anymore. It felt like being bombarded by strangers. I didn't know how to move or communicate.

I was so overwhelmed. My friends were there, and they were asking me things like "Phylecia are you okay? What happened?"

They knew something happened. They saw me one day, and then I was in the hospital three days later. They were coming up to me like they always had, but I was different.

A few weeks prior, I would come into Cracker Barrel, and everybody would be telling me their stories. I was all about it and all in.

Not anymore. I started shaking, and my heart was pounding. I was nervous and afraid.

I would go out to the floor where the tables were and feel stuck in place. I couldn't move.

It gives me chills and makes me tear up a little bit thinking about it.

I remember going back to the bathroom and crying, but I didn't know why or what was happening in my body. I was bent over the sink, hyperventilating and telling myself, *You can do this. You can do this.*

It was not a fun place to be.

I'm trying to describe this experience in terms you can understand; if you listen to the second episode of my podcast, you'll hear the true gravity. Here's an analogy: Imagine you had been a runner your entire life. You ran track in high school. You loved to run marathons. It is where you fucking thrived. Then one day you wake up, and you're paralyzed. The thing you were famous for doesn't work any longer. The thing you knew the most, the thing that you were most confident in, the thing you loved—it's no more.

That's what this was like. The thing I was most confident in, the thing I loved, the thing I was famous for was my personality—my bubbly, fun, outgoing, happy self who loved to talk to everyone. I loved to walk into work and dance with Allie. I loved to laugh with all the cooks and have friends over after work.

My only skill in life was talking to people. It was being social and making others laugh and feel good.

That was gone. I didn't know that I had gone through trauma, that I would lose my identity and have to start over from scratch with no sense of self to help me.

That day back at work, I came out of the bathroom trying to get my shit together. I had just been crying and shaking in the bathroom. One of the cooks saw me come out; he and I were the best of pals. He was always so happy, and we'd hug and laugh every day when we were both working. When he saw me come out, it was as if he saw a different person. I couldn't even look at him, because I would start crying again. I was heartbroken that he saw me like this. He said, "Phylecia! What's wrong girl? Be happy!" I didn't know what to say. I tried to smile, but tears welled up in my eyes, and I had to walk away.

My friend Noelle saw me. We made eye contact, and she knew something was wrong. She motioned to me, and we went back to the freezer. (The freezer is where we would go if we were either stressed or about to cry, because it would freeze our tear ducts, and then we wouldn't cry. Being a server is tough.)

Noelle was amazing because she had been there during the manic episode, and she was so good about being empathetic. She looked me in the eye and asked, "Phylecia, what's wrong? What is going on?"

"I don't know. I don't know. I don't know," I responded, panicked and upset.

I was breathing hard. I couldn't catch my breath. I started crying and said, "I can't handle this anymore." I was nervous, fearful, and anxious all at once.

Noelle said, "I'll take care of your tables. You just go home. I've got you."

So I dipped.

At that moment, I saw that life as I'd known it was over.

That was the fall.

As I write this, I am tearing up to even go back there. I don't think about this time a lot because it's not a fun place to be. When I'm in it like this, I remember that girl and I just feel so bad for her. I know there are people out there struggling all the time just like this.

And they don't have a path. They don't have somebody to tell them, "It's okay. This is just part of it. You're gonna get through it, we can build back."

That day at work was when my life came crashing down. That realization is a lot bigger than you might think, because my personality was gone.

I was so scared. Nobody told me what was going to happen or what to expect. My doctor didn't say, "Phylecia, listen. You are bipolar. You just had a manic episode. This is what just happened. This is what's going to happen. The natural progression of a manic episode is depression. Your depression is going to hit you, and this is what you need to expect."

It was like I was just going into the world exposed and had no idea what emotions were hitting me.

I was crippled.

It's not just about being depressed. It's not just about having a manic episode. It's not just about having to move out of my apartment because I couldn't pay my bills anymore. It's not about the fact that I was dependent on my parents. That's on-the-surface shit.

It's about how I did not know how to *be me* anymore. **I didn't know how to be Phylecia.**

I was not who I thought I was.

That realization was heartbreaking. *Oh my God.*

I have to lead up to this, because I'm going to start crying again.

The heartbreaking part was thinking—because I didn't know what else to think—that my entire life, my entire personality, and my entire persona that I was famous for were all just a lie. I believed really, I'd just been manic my whole life.

That was not true, but I did not know it at the time.

I still have an amazing personality. Yes, I am bipolar. But your diagnosis is not who you are. It's just a part of who you are.

But I did not know that.

I lost my sense of self. I lost my communication skills. I didn't know how to smile anymore. I didn't know how to laugh anymore. I didn't know how to socialize anymore.

The joy was gone.

I would look at other people and just feel sad. I was stuck in place, raw and exposed. I asked myself, *Why did this happen to me? This is not fair.* After I felt sad, I got angry.

Why do I have to take medicine to be okay? Why do I have to go to the psychiatrist and the therapist? Why did my parents have to go through this and why did my sister and friends see all that—why? Why did this happen to me? I'm a good person. This isn't right.

I was anxious, fearful, and sad, on a loop.

I remember having the feeling, *Is this it? Is this my life now?*

That is despair.

How do you deal with life when you have lost who you thought you were?

One of my friends shared something with me that she should have kept to herself. She said one of our other friends said, "Phylecia will never be the same."

Phylecia will never be the same. Can you imagine hearing that?

Given the state I was in, it still pisses me off to this day that she felt the need and had the audacity to tell me one of my friends said that.

But hearing it solidified the idea in my head. *He's right. It's over. I will never be Phylecia again.*

I'm never going to be the Phylecia they knew. I'm never going to be able to be cool and funny and have fun. Why would they be friends with me anymore?

One day I was at Cracker Barrel, before I quit for the second time. I worked the morning shift. My managers knew something happened, just not exactly what.

I had always been happy, dancing, and laughing. One of my managers could tell, obviously, that I was not smiling anymore. I went around flatlined, and he said to me, "Phylecia, what's wrong with you?"

"What . . .?" I replied.

He said, "Are you ever going to smile again?"

Just getting hit in the face one time after another.

On the worst day of my life, I woke up with severe depression. I was crying and felt like I couldn't move. Nothing had happened, but everything had happened. My mom was trying to console me but didn't know what to do. "Make it stop! Make it stop!" I pleaded.

It was like someone had died, or I was in physical pain. I felt a wave of depression and pure anxiety, and I could not get out of it. Then I experienced the next phase: I stopped crying and completely flatlined, with no emotion.

We made an emergency appointment with my psychiatrist.

When I got there, I was the most desperate I had ever been. I was looking—praying—for someone to tell me, "Phylecia, it's okay. We're going to get through this. I'm going to help you."

I went to him in my hour of need, and I asked him, "Is this it? Is this me now? Was my whole personality just a lie, a figment of a manic brain?"

His response: "Maybe."

Shatter.

My life crumbled at that moment. It was like a slow-motion movie, thinking about my past life, seeing pictures in my head of myself laughing, knowing how great my life was. Now all of that was fading into the background. Now I was this sad shell of the person I once was—someone with no confidence or self-esteem. Someone who felt laid bare and uncomfortable. Someone who would never be who they once were. I didn't know how to function anymore.

I was hoping and praying that he would say, "No, Phylecia, this is just depression. This is just the cycle. Your brain went through some mad trauma. We're going to get you through it."

And that's why I do what I do.

Depression is like being completely numb and so sad for no reason whatsoever.

You can *feel* depression. For instance, right now, I feel light and normal. I can move around. I can speak freely and with ease.

When you're depressed, you can feel the cloud and the shadow come over you. It feels like there is a weight, a ton of bricks on you—you feel dragged down. You cannot move the right way. You can't speak the right way. You can't get out of bed. You have to talk yourself into daily tasks. Everything seems impossible, and the depression tells you that you can't do anything.

It seems like we are diagnosed with this thing and are supposed to just know how to navigate it. That would be like never watching or playing football in your life and then walking out onto the Super Bowl field, with Andy Reid screaming at you to run the ball.

That's what it felt like: clueless, bare, and afraid.

Takeaways

At this time in my life, the missing piece was hope. I had no path or yellow brick road to follow. I didn't even understand my own diagnosis. After I had been through this trauma, the fall happened when I couldn't move or communicate like I had for my entire life.

I didn't know how to *be me* anymore.

I felt shattered and broken.

Chapter 6
My Parents' Strength

"Where there is no struggle, there is no strength."
—Oprah Winfrey

Now that you understand how far I fell, I want to talk about the climb back up. Hopefully by reading this, it won't take you as long as it took me to get out of the hole I found myself in.

I was no longer the social butterfly I'd once been. This new girl had an amount of social anxiety that's hard to measure. I didn't know how to spell the word "anxiety" before this. Before, I surrounded myself with people who were "above me" in terms of their successes or their career paths, but that was okay because I knew who I was. I surrounded myself with people all the time. Now the thought of simply going to the movies with my mom made my hands shake and heart pound.

I was nervous to leave the house, to be out in the open. I needed to feel safe. The only way I felt safe was being with my mom and dad. It was tough for my dad because usually he was the one with all the good quotes, all the positive vibes, all the life experiences, all the helpful feedback. But now? He didn't know what to say. He didn't know how to give me the kind of support I needed. As Elsa says in *Frozen II*, this was like going into the unknown.

I always loved my mom. We had a great relationship after high school. I was a true-blue bitch as a teenager, but we had come a long way since. She was the one I would learn to mirror, while my dad was the one I listened to.

There was one day when I was feeling sad and pitying myself, and I cried, telling my mom, "I just feel like a stupid little kid who can't leave her parents' side. I feel so stupid." My mom wasn't so good with words, but she didn't need to be. I needed someone there to listen and help me feel peace. She didn't know what she was doing at the time—she probably still has no idea the impact she made on my life, and I will never be able to repay her.

I had to move on from my past life and learn how to walk again.

My life broke into a million little pieces.

The things I used to do in my life before the manic episode that brought me laughter and joy no longer felt available to me. I used to love to work out, to go to dinners with my girlfriends, to be out and about in the world.

I hadn't seen my friends in months. I would get invited places, but I would always say I couldn't and to please not give up on me. I had some friends who would come visit, even though I would tell them not to. (You know who you are, and I am forever grateful.)

It broke my heart to see pictures of my past life and my friends or to watch movies that used to make me laugh, because at the time, I believed I'd never live like that again. This was my new normal: living at home and being stuck like glue to my parents. It was also a blessing, because I needed to be carried, and I was lucky enough to have parents like this. I can't imagine feeling the way I did and not having people in my corner. I was one of the lucky ones, and don't think for a second that I'm not aware of that now. When I felt bad about living at home, my dad reassured me, "You can live here until the cows come home."

I would go to my room and cry at night because my past life was just that—in the past.

I felt anxious all the time. Anytime my parents went to work, I would think, *What do I do now? What am I going to do today?* I was scared to be alone.

I ended up getting a job at my dad's car dealership. That's what I needed at that time. I was close to him every day.

All I could do then was try to feel safe.

When I started at Shelbyville Chrysler, I would hide my brokenness, or try to. Feeling self-conscious and learning how to be in a social job and talk to people was difficult.

As the first year ended after my "episode," I did try to be social. I remember going to dinner with three other girlfriends. These girls were people I'd known for years. They were my inner circle. Before, I would have had a great time. This time? I had to make myself go.

When I went with them to Mark's Feed Store, a local barbecue place we used to go to all the time, I sat in the chair, wondering what they saw.

What do I look like right now? Can they see that I've changed? Am I boring?

All of their lives kept moving forward. My friend Danielle was a probation officer, on her way to becoming a police officer. My friend Carolyn was living her best life with her fiancé. My friend Katie was in school to become a nurse practitioner. All I could think was, *WTF am I doing here? My life sucks. I am nowhere near them. I don't deserve to be sitting here. I don't want to be sitting here hearing all this bullshit when my life has ended.*

I was sad, but also angry. I didn't understand why this had happened to me and nothing had happened to my peers. My peers had passed me by, and I was stuck. That's all I could think about. *I don't want to hear how great they are. I don't want them to see who I am now. What could I even say about myself?*

That's what hurt the most: "Phylecia, how are you?"

Well let's see, I went to the hospital because I had a manic episode. I can no longer pay my rent, so I moved back in with my parents. I can't leave the house most of the time, other than going to work, where my dad takes me every day. I don't know who I am anymore, and I've forgotten how to be happy or how to talk to people. I've gained forty pounds. I am on three different types of medication that make my hands shake. I had to get glasses because the side effects include blurred vision, along with weight gain, hair loss, hand tremors, and a plethora of other great things. I can't sleep without meds anymore. I cry most days and can't think of good times because it breaks my heart. Other than that—I'm great.

What in the actual fuck was I supposed to say? *Why the fuck did this happen to me, and you all are just fine and dandy?*

At the end of the day, I wondered, *WHY ME? WHY did this happen? I was a good person. I had a great life. I don't understand. This is bullshit.*

I was trying hard to act "normal." What even *was* normal now? I didn't know. When I wasn't sad, I was mad. I questioned why this had happened to me, because it wasn't fair. It wasn't fair that my life had stopped while others were happy. What was different about them compared to me?

I wanted the answers. I had none. I was in limbo.

I had been through what would become my trauma, but I had a job and did go back to school that next year, which was a big deal to me. I had amazing parents and friends. They may not have understood what I was going through, but they were there. That's more than a lot of people have on their best days. I should have been grateful for that. I wasn't. Gratitude would have been a great way to look at things, but I couldn't see it. I couldn't see that amid all this turmoil, I was still putting one foot in front of the other, no matter how fucked up that footprint looked after I had left it. I was still getting up and trying to do what was right, even though what was right didn't feel normal.

Thankfully, things did get a bit easier. Not easy, but I started to get out of the house more. My mom and I had a tradition every week. I had my little receptionist job, and I would go to school on Tuesdays and Thursdays.

Every Tuesday after school, my mom and I would go to Goose Creek Diner. It was a little diner in town that had the best fried green tomatoes and sauce you've ever tasted. It was perfect, because on Tuesdays the fried green tomatoes just happened to be half off, and it was five-dollar day at the movies. This outing became our thing for two years. I could look forward to going to our diner and then seeing a movie with my mom. It didn't matter what movie it was.

I cherish those years now because they were of great importance in carrying me and ultimately helping me come back.

The days at the diner when we would meet after school and go to the movies bring back happy memories. I remember feeling as if I was exhausted from having to be around people and seeing my mom at the diner was an instant feeling of relief and joy.

Thank you for ever and ever, Mom.

My mom and I would go to two, maybe three movies every week. She knew it was a way to get me out of the house. I lived for those days. She didn't focus on me too much, meaning she didn't show that she felt bad for me. She didn't show pity. She just lived and had me by her side.

During this time, my sister and I had a fallout. Ashley and I had been best friends through high school and up until my manic episode. She had a really hard time when I was in the hospital. Before I went in, I had done some things that scared her. She was only sixteen. Maybe it's my ego talking, but I think I was an anchor for her for a long time when she was growing up. I believe she looked up to me. When I went away to college in Utah when she was fourteen, the wheels began to fall off her wagon. She no longer had an older sister to look up to, because I was far away.

Not to say too much about my sister, but she started getting into some trouble. When I came back, we were still close, but it was only months later that I had the episode and things changed.

She kept her distance. When she needed me the most, I wasn't there for her. I couldn't be. I couldn't be there for myself, so how would I be there for someone else? She didn't understand, and she went away. My sister and I didn't speak for a year.

I'm not going to share the details here, but let's just say that she had a sour taste in her mouth, which was fair. We would get into fights, and things were said that I thought were unforgivable. But she was young, and she was hurt too. She had her own demons. She had her own battle she was fighting.

To say the least, we were broken.

I had dyed my hair dark brown—to match my soul most likely. I couldn't be blonde and vibrant anymore, because fuck that—I wasn't. I wore dark clothes, had dark hair, and had no style. I had gained forty pounds in less than six months. I had stretch marks and a huge face out of nowhere. Part of me was beginning to show again, though.

I was in the car with my mom on our way home from a movie, and I was driving. I like to drive. We stopped at a red light. There was a little girl, about five or six years old, looking out the window, and we made eye contact. I started rolling the window up and down at her, and she started laughing. She thought it was hilarious that someone was interacting with her in a silly window manner. That was a good feeling. I laughed; I felt warm and light.

I hadn't felt that way in a long time. It was almost like remembering the smell of your grandma's house when you haven't been there in a long time—nostalgic. *Wow*, I thought, *is this what it feels like to feel good?* I felt free, light, and airy. For a few seconds, there wasn't darkness over me.

Then of course when the light turned green, because I was being poor and pitiful, I immediately said, "I wish I felt like that more," which brought the mood right back down.

My parents carried me. I have a tattoo on my inner arm for them because without them, I don't know where I'd be. I would most likely be dead, or a homeless person talking to themselves while going through an endless manic episode.

Let's say too that all of this scared the shit out of them. I learned while writing this book how scared my parents were during my manic episode. Then they were heartbroken to see me the way I was after.

My dad said, "Yeah, there's no book on what to do if your daughter has a mental breakdown."

After everything was said and done, my dad got me out of my apartment lease but still had to pay for two months' rent because I had quit my job and then was in a hospital. They also had tons of medical bills—from UofL Hospital, the ambulance, and ten days at a mental health hospital—so you can imagine the financial strain.

On top of that, my mom accidentally gave the hospital the wrong insurance card. It was January, and she hadn't gotten her new card. During the craziness of all this, she made a human error and gave them the insurance card for the year before. That became a nightmare. The insurance companies rejected everything and wouldn't listen when my mom told them it was a physical mistake; the wrong insurance card was given, but we *did* have insurance. She called so many people and even wrote letters. They wouldn't listen. So my parents had to pay out of pocket for my care, which I am sure was close to $30,000, if not more. I had no idea until years later.

My parents are not made of money, so this was yet one more strain. But they never said a word about it in front of me. I never knew how stressed they were.

In my eyes, my parents were heroes, they were my saviors. Looking back, they didn't give advice—other than saying, "It's going to be okay," and my dad telling me to write down things to be grateful for. They didn't need to give a lot of advice, because they acted. My dad would give me things to do if I was feeling anxious. We would work out in the yard or in the garage.

My mom was my best friend. She would become my rock and the only person I ever wanted to be around on any given day—for years. She took this shit in stride, but she wouldn't tell you that. To this day, she would just say she had no idea what she was doing. But that woman somehow knew exactly what to do.

I was sad all the time, no emotion, no enthusiasm for anything. I wouldn't ever want to do anything. Getting out of the house was important but hard. I never wanted to leave, let alone take a shower or brush my hair. My mom would say, "Oh, come on, let's go. Get up, come on."

So I would get up with a sigh. *Ughhh* . . . I'd take a deep breath and say, "Okay." And wherever we went, I was a drag, but she didn't let that show. She just kept on living and made me live with her.

One day when we got out of the house, it was cold outside. We had gone out to breakfast, which was enough, but then she wanted to go to Walmart. I did not. I wanted to stay in the car, but she made me get out. She said, "Just come on, let's go." She didn't make a big fuss, just told me to get out of the car. My experience of life felt like it was in fragments. I couldn't look too far in the future, because right then, I just needed to get out of the car.

One moment at a time.

When I got out of the car, she got a cart, and it was windy. She was wearing her big, long, pink puffer coat, her hair was everywhere, and she was running in with her cart as the wind was blowing. She looked so silly. I chuckled a little to myself.

That was the first time in months that I had naturally smiled and laughed. I felt the cold air, and I felt like I could breathe again. I felt lighter and free.

I had felt so weighted down and dark, but in that moment, I felt okay for a second.

If I had stayed in the car like I wanted to, I wouldn't have chuckled to myself or felt like I could breathe again.

I will never forget that day. My mom has such a beautiful spirit—it is effortless. She had no idea what she did for me that day. I will remember that forever. As I write this, I am crying because I know my mom and dad were so worried and stressed, but I never saw it. I only saw them carry me, time and time again. I will spend my life paying them back. When I think about that time, I think about Celine Dion's song "Because You Loved Me." The lyrics could have been written from me to my parents.

Takeaways

At this point in the story, we're still in Stage 2 of the Bipolar Life Cycle—the aftermath, with guilt, blame, and self-pity. I was asking, "Why me?" I was angry and didn't understand why this had happened to me, but I was trying to climb out of it, little by little, day by day. I needed to feel safe, and I am so grateful I had my parents with me. I was one of the lucky ones.

Journal Interlude

On the following pages, you'll find entries from my journal during this time, so you can really feel where I was mentally. There's no better way to describe my experience than just sharing with you what I actually wrote. These entries are from February 2010, shortly after leaving The Brook.

(feb. 11, 2010)
•"episode": week of Jan. 6 – 8 2010.
•Ten Brooke: 10 days Jan thru Jan. 18th
got out Martin Luther King Day.
•going to my meetings ever since
last mtg is tom. feb. 12 2010.
I'm scared, I feel like I need those
meetings to stay sane. I was scared
today about the future (etc)
ppl / family what I would do if
my immediate family died →
I would mentally die. If I am ever
hooked up to a machine, not myself,
unable to speak → in misery.
please put me out of it. I would
much rather chill up north with
friends & family then down here
unable to do so. I love everyone
in my life right now. I feel on
the verge of crying a lot these
days because I honestly don't know
where I would be w/out the gospel,
Heavenly father, Jesus Christ, my
mom, my pop, my sister, my friends

[I cannot believe where my head was. Was I thinking I would never do cool shit again, so hopefully everyone remembers that? Were these suicidal thoughts? I don't know. Back to the journal entry . . .]

you know who & where you
are. stinnz, amanda, carolyn,
ashley, erica, shelby, jen, iah,
jordan, shane, bea, everyone
who has carried me this last
month, I will love forever.
I hope someone reads out of my
journal at my funeral.
try not to cry negatively at my
funeral; cry tears of joy. celebrate
my life and tell stories of all the
cool shit we did together. that's
what I will try my best to do
for you all. If you make it to
one of 2 parties in my life,
make one either my wedding,
or my funeral → and look you're
best! cuz ditto for you.
(snottin everywhere (interlude)
foot print prince → I am being
carried right now, not walking alone.
↳ it scares me because I dont know
what to do with myself.
♡ phylecia feb. 11, 2010 (at parents house)
8:04pm thurs.

Feb. 15 2010

I just had a breakdown and talked to my parents. Me crying, them telling me its going to be okay. This is about a weeks mark of me feeling depressed. I have never felt this way in my life. My dad told me to write a gratitude list of 20 to focus on the good things going for me instead of the bad. Here goes...

* Things I am thankful for today.

- my Dad
- my mom
- my sister
- my House
- my dogs
- missionaries
- The gospel
- my friends
- my family
- my Job
- the car I have
- 2 beds I can sleep in
- my mom being my best friend
- my dad being my [illegible] conscious
- my phone
- my clothes
- gym membership
- Carolyn
- Kristina
- Amanda
- my Boys
- my family
- everything else I may be forgetting at this time

[You can see there at the end I was grasping at straws but wanted to make it to twenty. Also, I was twenty-one years old, so some things were a little silly, but that's where I was.]

1/13 3:40 am I don't know why
I am awake... please help me go
to sleep. I pray for strength to go back
to sleep without my medication.
I am worried about everything - but not
anything. Please help me go back to
sleep is my only prayer right now....
I feel anxious & sick to my stomach &
coughing/sneezing. help!

•feb. 17, 2010.
I feel okay but a little anxious & scared to see my mom leave for work today. she has been with me for 3 whole days and I've depended on her. heavenly father please help me have strength.
↳ going to work today. Noelle called earlier & made me feel better for the time being. (Noelle rocks) good girl she is. Heavenly father please help our family. more than ever right now. we need you.
•feb. 18, 2010
I felt good last night after work. I wish I could feel like that all the time. Today I feel sad & I don't know what to do really, with myself. My dad & I spooned today like we used to when I was a kid. my mom goes to work at 3 @ today. what to do?
↳ my mom is about to leave for work, I'm gonna try to take a nap & then hang w/ my sister. [redacted]

- feb. 19, 2010
I have been out of the Brooke for a month now & only hope to get better from here.
me & my dad are hanging out today. He's gonna stay here w/me until about 3pm & I work at 5 so hopefully that will keep me occupied.
- feb. 20, 2010 - going to eat lunch w/ the missionaries. (weird!) but okay. I dont know if I should tell them about Ashley, I dont think I am.
↳ I did tell them.
- feb. 21, 2010
I'm going to church, ashley isnt.
- feb. 23, 2010
I had a good day today. I felt the same all day. not depressed, not hyper, but calm. I was able to chill. I hung out with Darian between 6-8 that helped with getting me out of the house. I think I'm feeling better today because we read & prayed last night w/ my dad

in the room. He loved it, just
doesn't know it yet. my mom & I
read tonight but my dad didn't.
thats okay - baby steps - I hope
we can have a miracle in this
family. we need one. either w/
[illegible] or my sister. as of today,

sad day. I just want it to go
back to normal. I did find out
today that we are going on vacation
for the first time in yearssss! I
am very excited about it. But
also nervous. But I think its
going to be exactly what our family
needs.

gratitude list

- my house - my car
- my family - my job
- my health - my friends.

feb. 24, 2010
good day today. slept alot, went to the gym and saw a movie (It's complicated) w/ my mom. It was really good. They smoked the reefer which made me miss it Ö I want to smoke! but its okay right? one day at a time. Thanks for everything heavenly father. I'll be back w/ more thoughts later!

• feb. 25, 2010
went to my 1st therapy session today. I like her, I think thats what I want to do when i get older. I feel okay today, but boring. I want my fun, personality back.

• feb. 27, 2010
Its saturday and i had the day off. i slept til noon, slept some more, worked out, showered, slept some more, and now I'm going to dinner w/ katie Howard + leah oppy. I hope I put on my happy face and they cant

tell that I'm not the same as
when they saw me last. I'm blah
today, but more sad because I am
showing nothing, no emotion.
I miss my mom and she's just at
work.

Chapter 7
What to Expect after a Manic Episode

Your Number One Job Is to Become Stable

Alrighty, let's get into what I was never told: what the hell to expect *after* a manic episode.

First, you must know that what just happened put your brain, your body, and most likely your friends and family through something traumatic.

I didn't think what I went through was trauma, but it was.

I was never told how significant this was or what the natural progression would be.

A manic episode in bipolar I is followed by depression. The natural progression of mania is depression. You can bet that if you feel great and you're manic, the next step—whether minutes, days, or weeks later—is you're going to be depressed.

It's a wild concept too. Your mind in mania tells you things like: *You are the best person who has EVER lived. You can do anything. You're the king of the world. You're pretty much God. You can do it ALL. You are gorgeous. You have all the money in the world to help everyone.*

Then the fucked-up part is depression is the total opposite. In minutes, your brain tells you this: *You are a fucking loser. You are fat. No wonder you have no friends—you don't deserve friends.* Remember, depression lies. *You shouldn't even get out of bed today—what's the point? What's the point of life if we all die anyway? You can't do anything; you're an idiot for thinking that you can. You might as well just stay here.* (And, as you might imagine, it can get worse—much worse.)

It's not just "Yay, I'm happy!" and then "Oh no, I'm sad." It's extremely, dangerously dramatic.

Years later, when I was ultimately pretty level, the highs and lows would still come and go. I would be on cloud nine, go to the gym, and feel great. I wasn't experiencing a manic episode, but it was when mania would pop in. My brain in this state would feel amazing, like, *Girl, you GOT life. You are THE shit.* But the energy would deplete, and then my brain would tell me,

Yeah, right, you're not the shit—you're a piece of shit. Go home and stay there. You're a loser.

When I would feel like this, the energy I had moments before would exhaust me to think about. *OMG, how was I just jumping around in my car so happy a second ago, and now I'm back to flatlined?*

It's like you must start from scratch in this progression to get to center again.

For me, I'd feel good about where I was in my life. I'd think, *Okay, you've got this now.* Then, depression would come and totally throw me off kilter.

So, it's not fluid. It's stop and go, stop and go, like football. Feel great: *I can do this.* Then: *No you can't you're stupid.* Then: *Okay, wait I've gotta get out of this. Okay, I'm getting out of it—now where was I?*

Those ups and downs will come and go through your Bipolar Life Cycle, but here's the great part: that doesn't happen to me like it used to at all.

I haven't had highs and lows like that in many years. And don't get me wrong: I don't wait for the other shoe to drop, but I know that shadow is there and could attach to me any minute.

Here's the difference: I now know exactly what I do if it does.

When you work this cycle, the highs and lows aren't so dramatic. If they do come in, you've got tools. Then they may not come again for years on end.

We are playing the long game. If you want to make a comeback from any kind of trauma, it is a marathon, not a sprint.

I can look through my own curve. Sometimes in life, you must anticipate what is coming down the road. When my dad taught me how to drive, he told me, "Look through the curve so you can see and be prepared for what's coming." The same applies here: I have a plan for this year, but I do not want to overwhelm myself. I know that if I get overwhelmed and start doing too much, mania can sink in, then depression. And I do not have time for that.

My point is this: fourteen years later, sure, I'm doing well—but I do not disrespect the disorder that I have. I know it's there, and I respect that. But I also don't accept its limitations. I fight against that shit to this day and will forever.

Doing so has just gotten easier. It is second nature.

Make stability and survival number one, because when you do, it becomes *normal* to take care of your needs. Get familiar with the disorder. Understand it and how it affects you, along with the solutions and tools available to you.

Once you have that down, you move on. You don't want to be in this constant cycle. You are not *just* bipolar—you are a person who has so much to give. Bipolar is a part of the game you play, but you can win that game.

Hitting you with yet another metaphor: Think about trying to run a marathon. You don't just wake up one day and say, "Huh, I'm gonna run a marathon tomorrow."

A few years after I got back to myself, I wanted to run a half-marathon. It's 13.1 miles, and I couldn't run for thirty seconds straight. Guess what I did?

I got an app that did cycles. First it was thirty seconds on, thirty seconds off. Then I moved to one minute on, one minute off. Then two minutes on, one minute off. I kept doing that, and weeks later, I was able to run for five minutes straight. Now mind you, that's not even one mile.

It took me about twelve minutes to run one mile. A half-marathon is 13.1 of those. But I booked the race. I had sixteen weeks to whip myself into shape.

I looked through the curve.

Then I scheduled a 10K first, which was twelve weeks away. A 10K is about six miles.

My first milestone was coming.

I kept working with this app, and I got to where I could run two miles nonstop. Are you getting my point yet? I kept going.

I completed the 10K without stopping, though it was a *crawl* of a jog, if that. Women in their sixties who were power walking were passing me. But I did it.

The 13.1 miles were four weeks away. That was *tough*. I was one of the last to finish. They were opening the damn roads, and I was still going. My legs were lead by the end. By mile eleven, I thought there is no freakin' way, dude. I kept going. I was on a competitive swim team in high school, but I was totally out of shape leading up to this race, and my legs even after swim meets had never been this sore. I felt like I could not walk, let alone jog or run.

I did stop to walk, and then I'd jog. Then I'd walk again, and so on. But I finished that damn race with so much pride. I had the biggest smile on my face. I was lucky enough to have my parents there to see me at the end.

It was something I wanted to do, and I did it. Slow and steady did not win the race, but it sure as shit finished it.

Working out for that race was unfamiliar, hard, and tiring in the beginning. Then it became my normal. It became what I did.

In sticking to it, I was able to run a race, gain confidence, and lose a couple pounds. It wasn't about the race itself; it was the climb. It's what happened after: confidence. I felt independent again because I did it totally on my own. I didn't have a friend or a running partner. It was my thing, and I wanted to do it for myself.

Think of that story like your Bipolar Life Cycle. It's hard. It's the hardest thing I've done in my life, to come back after what happened in 2010. It challenged my entire being and self. I lost who I was, but somehow, I knew I had to keep going.

When I kept putting one foot in front of the other, it became natural. Then I was able to add on what I enjoyed doing.

I was able to run that race, I was able to get my own beautiful apartment, and I was able to go on a three-week solo road trip—but not before I got centered and tried to stay there.

The point is, after a manic episode you may lose your sense of self—for a time.

You have to know what mania is, how you feel when mania sets in, and what you are going to do to come down. But if you plan enough, if you set your life with intention, you can run this marathon.

Never let anyone tell you suffering is just the way it is. There is always a road to walk down.

After a manic episode, you should be researching holistic approaches to getting your mind and body level. What kinds of medications are going to work for you? Find the right support team, doctors, and routines. We don't find a routine for the good days; we have a routine for the bad ones.

First things first: getting level and staying centered.

This is just like an addict's job when they're getting sober. Their number one job is staying sober. That's it. Not family, not church, not work—it's sobriety. Because if they are not *sober*, nothing else mentioned before is possible to keep, love, or do effectively.

It's important to give the disorder the respect it deserves, but that doesn't mean we don't fight.

In this stage, it's survival. We aren't worried about dreams and goals yet. It's how to feel *okay* every day. This is the hardest thing you'll do other than trauma relating to loss, abuse, etc. This is it.

Getting level on meds and finding the right doctors is a process. It took two full years to find the right meds and dosages. You are playing the long game, but I promise you, if you keep playing, you will come out like Tom Brady winning his seventh Super Bowl.

Bipolar is an explanation, but *it is not an excuse.*

We cannot live our lives using this excuse all the time. We cannot affect others, or treat others like shit, without taking responsibility. We cannot think the sun rises and sets on our ass. A diagnosis is not an excuse for bad behavior. It is our *duty* take responsibility; no one else is coming to save us.

Part of this is going to be dealing with the side effects of meds. It was for me. I gained forty pounds in about six months. I not only hated myself because of depression and what happened but also because I hated my body. I didn't know who I was, and I didn't recognize myself for a long time.

But I did know this: my priority was not my physical body—it was my brain. It was not wanting to feel shitty every day, and not becoming manic again. All I was concerned about was coming out of that cycle and figuring out how to breathe again.

After that manic episode, I began living my life so something like that never happened again. You must do the same.

Later, you'll progress and develop more skills. But right after an episode and diagnosis, your only concern is stability and what you do daily to get through it, feel okay, and stay safe.

If you have kids and responsibilities, that's a priority—but if you're not stable, you're not going to be who you need to be for those kids. Make your mental health the top priority while parenting your children. You take responsibility for them just as much as you fight for your own mental health and stability.

If you have the means or chance, make sure you have health insurance. If you're on meds, you do not want to skip prescriptions because you can't afford them. When you have health insurance, your therapist and psychiatrist appointments won't be hundreds of dollars.

You've gotta think about this stuff, y'all. I hear way too much, "Well, I can't afford to go to the therapist," or "I'm too busy to go to the therapist."

You do whatever you need to do to be able to afford to invest in your own mental health and stability. Period.

You find the time. You find the dollars. Things like psychiatry don't have to be every week. I went to my psychiatrist once a month, then every three months, then once a year. But in the beginning, having the visits you need is so important in coming back.

Takeaways

Stability first: Get prescribed meds and get level on meds. Find the right doctors. Have the right trusted team in place.

Do something that will make you feel productive at least one time each day. It could literally be taking out the trash and having to walk to the garbage can. That's how simple this shit is right now. It could be painting your nails. It could be changing the lightbulb that's been needing a replacement for six months.

Do that on repeat as many times as it takes until the clouds begin to lift. And they will.

Chapter 8
Coping and Solutions

"There is hope, even when your brain tells you there isn't."

—John Green

There are two types of people out there: the ones who have a problem, lie down, and blame others—and the ones who immediately look for the solution. Let's be the latter guy.

Your personality will come back—slowly, but it will. And once it's back, hot damn, there is nothing better.

I hope you have some hope. That's what this is about. It's understanding what's to come and the progression of bipolar, but also how to get out of this shit quickly.

At this stage, you don't move on to real growth until you've solidified the coping mechanisms and the solution to getting through your day-to-day with this disorder. When your mental health becomes second nature, *then* you begin to figure out who you want to be.

My journey took about five years to come 100 percent back.

If it's been a year or more since your initial diagnosis and you feel you're still flailing and do not have a day-to-day routine for your mental health in place (i.e., medication, a trusted therapist, a psychiatrist, and a sense of leveling out on medications), you need to go back to the basics: What is your routine? What are your solutions? What kind of support do you have?

After that, you'll begin to see sunshine come back and spots of your personality—your old self.

You need to take things like cleanliness and hygiene seriously. If your house is a mess and dirty, you will feel like a mess and dirty. If your body is stinking and your hair is greasy, that's feeding depression. I know it's hard. I know everything in your being is telling you to stay in bed, not to shower, not to brush your teeth. You might be thinking, *I don't have the energy to get up and put the dishes away.*

Make yourself. Unless you literally have no legs or can't walk, you can do this. People say, "I can't, I can't." Actually, you can. But you must *make* yourself do the thing.

Baby steps, but cleanliness is vital. When you get out of the shower, you're not going to be magically happy, but it helps. And I bet you, for about ten minutes you weren't just sitting there thinking about how shitty life is. You were thinking, *Okay, I've gotta rinse my hair now.*

Your mind was distracted. That's what all of this becomes. You have to do things so that your brain and mindset can shift from stewing on "I hate myself" to saying, "Okay, I'm doing a thing, and that's where my brain power is going."

Get started, even if it's just ten minutes a day. Progress, not perfection. Then you'll be able to add on to that.

For me, years two and three were about taking control of the diagnosis.

A big factor in your success is your support team, but also being part of that team. Helping others will come in time.

Once I became mentally stable and started seeing my personality come back bit by bit, I started doing things I used to enjoy, like taking baby steps in hanging out with friends and going to the gym. Doing things, you know will make you feel good is just a step to get you to your next pivotal moment.

So how to cope with bipolar? Well, first you must understand the disorder and the progression. You must know what type of bipolar you are: I or II? Then you learn the natural progression of mania is toward depression.

You then figure out what the trigger for your onset was. For me, in hindsight, I see I was doing all the things, and that frenetic activity progressively got worse. I had to stop myself anyway, and it turns out I was bipolar I, so mania was a natural event.

I now know that if I'm doing a lot, I need to focus on maintaining a center of gravity. Pay attention to your sleep and your meds. You need to look through the curve and know what's possible down the road.

It is not only a possibility that you're going to wake up manic or depressed; it is a *probability*. There's a difference. Knowing that—and being okay with it—represents a pivotal moment.

You don't need to be scared—if you're prepared. I tell my nephew that all the time. I talk to him about what happens in an emergency and what the plan is. I say, "We don't have to be scared if . . ." and he responds, "We're prepared," with a roll of the eyes.

But it's true. You face this shit head-on. You know you're bipolar, and like I said in the beginning of this book, you first must *recognize* that you have a disorder. Then you must accept it: *Okay, I have this thing that I need to deal with.* If you aren't accepting of the fact that you have a disorder in the first place, then you're not ready for coping mechanisms. You must start by acknowledging there's a problem.

I think a lot of the time people are embarrassed. They don't want to admit that they have a mental disorder. As a result, it's tempting to live in denial. But here's the truth: if you're living in denial or don't want to take care of it, and you try to ignore it—it will be something that continues to derail your life and the people closest to you time and time again. You will make people disappear because *you* are not taking care of your business.

So, accept you have a problem. Understand that problem, its definition, and how it relates to you.

Remember, getting level and stable is *numero uno.* We know what those mechanisms look like.

Once you find stability, and you find a way to live daily, distracting your mindset enough will move you toward really being able to rebuild your own foundation. We are focused on ourselves in this phase. We do have other priorities like jobs, families, relationships, and so on, but we are number one right now.

Solutions for me at this time included needing to:

- Understand how to distract myself.
- Understand my own diagnosis, triggers, and onsets.
- Find the right medications and doctors.
- Have responsibility.
- Feel a sense of purpose.
- Identify what brings me confidence and makes me feel independent.

I want you to write those things down. Responsibility and distraction, independence and confidence—they go hand in hand. Because when you have that foundation in place, and you know those things about yourself, then you can start to move forward. That's when the change happens.

Helping others is a distraction and will absolutely help you move forward. A huge solution for me is knowing I have someone I can go help. It's not "I know who I can talk to when I feel bad," though of course that's important—but what's more important is completely distracting yourself when it comes to depression. If you're helping someone else, your focus is *them*, not you.

I say you are the focus of your own stability, and of course you are, but the bigger idea here is that it is not all about you in life itself. It can't be. You've got to find your own solutions; no one else will do that for you. The only one who can save you is you, playa. So let's go.

You cannot think your way out of depression. Your mind got you there, and it cannot get you out. Thinking, "*Man, I'm so depressed—I need to get out of this,*" isn't helpful. You must distract yourself from that mindset. The more you focus elsewhere on someone or something else for a long period of time, the more the clouds will begin to lift.

Have you ever heard that "back in the day," when people were on farms and working physically every day to survive, no one had depression? Maybe that's true, and maybe it's not, but there's truth in it. They literally didn't have time to be depressed because they were focused on their own survival. Same methodology—if you have "social anxiety" and you stay home all the time, you're forever going to have social anxiety, because you aren't working on any kind of progress or solution.

Make sense?

You have a choice, right here, right now: you either take responsibility for yourself and for your life and start the fight, *or* you stay exactly where you are. On the second path, you blame everyone else for your problems, you feel bad for yourself, and life isn't fair.

Yeah, life is not fair. But what are you going to do about it? Make the choice.

I read a book by Mike Bayer called *One Decision*, about making one decision today that will change the rest of your life. It just takes one decision. That decision could be staying in bed and feeding depression—or letting yourself fly off the handle into mania and never caring enough to solve what's going on.

Or you could decide to figure out what you're going to do to get out of depression and come down from mania.

For me, distraction from depression and mania means calming my body or discharging energy by working out. It becomes that simple.

In the beginning, you're going to have to work hard on it every single damn day. Keep trudging forward. Sometimes your trudge will be so basic: *How do I get out of bed today? How do I get myself to work? How do I make sure I stay calm?*

Later, it will be: *Okay, great, I can get out of bed, but what can I do that will make me feel productive?* You'll be able to focus on cleanliness again and organization. Make a list of what you want to conquer within the week and find a way to get it done.

When you feel productive and clean, and when you can distract your brain, productivity and distraction become your solutions. The actual strategies inside of these two solutions will change over time, but you start with the basics.

Actual strategies I use: Get outside, and get clean, fresh air. Go to a friend's house who has kids and hang out with their kids. If you don't have friends, go into your community and figure out how you can be around someone who needs help. Get involved with a church if that's your thing—at the very *least*, church is a community. Get involved in Al-Anon. There are so many people in those types of atmospheres who are trying to get better. Get involved with people who are trying to get better too—not people who are okay with feeling shitty. There's a difference. GO HELP SOMEONE ELSE. Life is not all about you! For a time, you are in survival mode, but at some point, you've got to distract your brain enough for the clouds of depression to lift. Who needs your help?

Exercise and eat healthy. This is huge for coping and solutions. I know that a direct trigger of depression is when I eat like shit, I feel like shit. When I feel crappy about what I've put into my body, I become lazy and lethargic. That can then bring on depression.

I know that when I'm doing a lot, I can easily slip into mania. I stay on my meds and get enough sleep. I schedule time to relax. I schedule sauna and float visits so I can concentrate on being calm.

Meditation and journaling will help keep you centered and calm as well. Do that every single day. Make this a practice for gratitude, mood levels, and daily check-ins—later you can use it for setting goals as well.

Work on prayer. You don't have to be religious to pray. Praying does multiple things: it builds hope, it gets your worries and gratitude out in the open, and it makes you feel less alone. It also distracts your brain for a few minutes.

Remember, all of this is in the realm of preparation and intentionality. You must come in every single day doing these things to stay centered.

You cannot get so busy in life that you stop doing what made you stable. Just because you're stable for five minutes or five years doesn't mean you can take for granted that you will continue to be.

Again, the fucked part and the beauty of bipolar is that we can get in and out of shit quickly.

Being happy won't last forever, so live in that moment for as long as possible, because you aren't guaranteed it in the next minute. But if we work to stay there as long as we can, those happy moments will last longer.

Know that the bad doesn't last. It goes hand in hand with the good. Live inside the great moments, because you don't know what's going to happen tomorrow. But the bad moments can leave quickly if we want them to.

When you feel bad, remember what you did the time before to get out of it. One more mechanism: when you feel bad, do something you know makes you laugh or calms you down. A diversion is what we're looking for here. Do something that you know will bring you joy, even if it doesn't at that moment.

When you begin to work on these things, the next time you feel depressed, you'll be able to say, "I mean, I got out of it before—I just have to do it again."

I've done it before; I just have to do it again.

Let's fight the *right* battle so that we can move on and bipolar is just the game we play.

When mania and depression come on, you need to know how you feel and what your triggers are so that you can prevent being triggered in the first place. You must know how you *feel* when mania or depression comes on so that you can identify it quickly. We want to immediately look for the solution so that we don't stay there too long and get lost.

It's almost like water on the stove that you want to warm but not boil. You must pay attention to the water, ensuring it's steady and where you want it to be, and you need to know when to turn off the burner or move the pot *before* it boils. If it begins to boil, it takes longer to cool down, and it could splash over the top and burn you.

It's the constant fight of staying steady, consistent, balanced, and centered so that the pot doesn't boil over. But if it does get too hot, and you did fuck up a little and let it boil, *what are you going to do to cool it down?* That's the question.

It's not: *Hey, how do I touch this water that's boiling? Should I wear a glove to see if the water is still hot? Should I just be pissed that I let it spill over and walk away and accept it?*

Nope, we figure out the best next step to get that water where we want it.

Ask yourself the right questions.

The wrong question: *How do I stop spending all my money when I'm manic?*

The right question: *How can I get out of mania, and what is my best next step to get centered?*

No, you don't want to spend all your money when you're manic, but you've got to focus on the solution to getting out of this thing instead of accepting it, staying there, and trying to "treat the side effects."

You need to know how to lower the temperature without bringing yourself too far down. There's a fine little line between mania and depression. What's going to bring you back up from depression? What if you have anxiety—how can you get out of that anxiety or that anxiety attack? I have plans, strategies, and tools for all these situations, because I know it's probable that I could wake up tomorrow in that state, and I don't have time for it.

We are stronger than this disorder. Do not bow down to it.

My friend and I were talking about how she struggles with anxiety and depression. Her therapist has a good metaphor. In his office, he has a picture of a white wolf and a black wolf. He said to her, "So let me ask you this: If you feed the black wolf all the time, and you starve the white wolf, who's going to be stronger?"

She said, "Well, the black wolf."

"Exactly," he replied.

The black wolf is depression. If you feed depression, it's going to be stronger than you. You are the white wolf. You are just you—you come out of the womb just as strong as the black wolf is. Yes, it's there, and it can pop up on your ass. But if you starve out the depression, if you don't fuck with it, if you say to the black wolf, "Here it is—I got you, dude," you cultivate your own strength. I've learned depression is like a person I don't want around. I say to myself, *here you are, motherfucker. And I am done. I am not dealing with you for more than four hours.* It's down to a science.

Feed that white wolf. What I mean by that is take care of your business every freaking day. If you do, you are going to become untouchable.

It's hard to get out of depression and to do something about it. But you know what's harder? Being in a constant state of depression—so choose your hard.

This is all intentionality and living a centered, balanced life so that we don't swing so far on the emotional and bipolar pendulum.

Takeaways

You cannot think your way out of depression. The battle is all about physical distraction. You must stay centered daily. When mania or depression hit, know in advance what you are you going to do about it. What helps you stay calm and sleep? Which medications keep you level? How will you keep clean and productive? All of this will become second nature, but that doesn't mean you set it and forget it. You must ensure you are centered daily, in order to move on to bigger and better things.

Rock on.

Part III
Rebuilding the Foundation

Chapter 9
Learning to Breathe Again

"Don't stay down too long. Don't you waste your life in them dark rooms by yourself. Don't do it."
—Jennifer Lewis

I want to share the story of Riley. She was a huge contributor to my ability to care about something or someone else, a being other than myself.

As I mentioned before, a couple months after I quit Cracker Barrel, I got a job as the receptionist for the service department at the car dealership where my dad worked.

That job was exactly what I needed at that time in my life. My dad worked a couple feet away from me. I started working there a few months after leaving The Brook, sometime in 2010.

Part of the journey toward healing is identifying what you need to make just the present moment better. For me, safety was the most important piece. If you're not lucky enough to have parents to catch you, find support elsewhere and a place you feel safe too. (Then you can move on to bigger and better things down the road.)

There was an animal shelter nearby, and they brought some puppies to the dealership one day. This is when I met Riley. She was the only brindled female puppy amid black-and-white brothers. My dad brought her back to my office, and I was hooked. I couldn't think of a name though. She was sporty, like me—so her name couldn't be too girly. At first, I named her Lacey, but now thinking of that name in association with her makes me want to throw up. She wasn't a Lacey. When I brought her home, she started to show her crazy personality and her tomboy queen ways—then I found it: Riley. Riley was my girl and my best friend.

As I write this, she is gone now, but I want to tell you all about her and how she helped me become *me* again.

Riley gave me something to care about other than myself and my bipolar disorder. I had to make sure she was cared for, fed, and potty-trained. I also had to train her, because the girl was insane. She had so much damn energy—she was like me in my manic state. It was awesome. Riley would come in from outside like a Tasmanian devil.

She was a pit bull–boxer mix, brindled and beautiful. She was athletic and sporty, but feminine too. She always smelled good. She had a little white spot on her nose and one on each of her paws. She would run full blast from outside, fly over my dad on the couch, run around the room seventeen times, and finally lie down when she was ready. Cesar Millan would be very disappointed, but that was Riley. We did end up giving her lessons, and she did great.

Not only did having Riley by my side help me, but she was also a light. I don't think I even knew that at the time. I just thought she was my dog and my best friend, and taking care of the dog is what you do when you have one, but she brought me back to life.

That chick didn't give a shit if I was happy, sad, fat, skinny, flatlined, crying—she loved me every single day. She didn't care what I looked like or who I was the day before. She was the heartbeat and the rhythm I needed. She could look so deep into my eyes and touch my soul. She slept in my bed, right up against my back like my pillow.

As the months and years went on, Riley was always there. She was a constant. I took so much pride in Riley. She was the first puppy I ever raised. I was hers and she was mine. She was a dog, but I felt like she knew who I was.

Riley helped me learn how to walk on my own again. As we grew up together, we grew a little older. She has since passed, but my sister made me five canvases of photos of Riley and me as well as Riley and my nephew together. I can look at Riley every single day and remember her spirit—and what she got me through.

Riley gave me responsibility. I had to care about a being other than myself. That was her most important gift to my recovery. I had a reason to get out of the house, to go take walks and ensure she had a great life.

Everything was not just about me and being depressed.

Through this responsibility came confidence. I was confident in my dog and what I had trained her to do. This, in turn, gave me a sense of pride and independence I hadn't felt in a long while. She also gave me so much joy.

There's the pivotal moment: through raising Riley, I had a sense of independence, confidence, and joy in my life again. It made me care about somebody other than myself.

There are many people struggling more than we are. There is a dog somewhere who needs a home. The mentality of "I need to distract myself and go help someone else or gain a responsibility" is where we want to be.

Note: I'm not saying go have a kid. I'm not saying go get a dog if you don't have the means to take care of the dog. Use your common sense as much as you can. But go out in your community, volunteer, and **help somebody else**.

I will never forget Riley and what she did for me.

Learning how to breathe again had a long road ahead. Taking care of Riley helped me get out of the house more often. I slowly started to try and be around my close friends.

A nod to friends who were there at the time:

Two of my friends were Nick and Krystina. They were a couple. I had known Krystina since middle school and Nick for about eight years. I found that I was able to hang out with them; they were in my comfort zone.

My good friends Ian, Carolyn, Katie, and Shane never wavered. When I didn't want to go out, they came to me. Shane took me out one night years later and danced with me and made me feel like a princess. Katie and Carolyn came over though it was tough for them to see me the way I was, and they never gave up. Once Ian called me, and I said I couldn't hang out. He came over and picked me up, as he knew I needed to get out of the house. I lay on his lap, and we watched a movie. I will never forget these moments, and I hold them close to my heart every day.

Do not discount people you can lean on in these times of need. I know how truly lucky I am to have these people in my corner. If you don't, you can always *always* find someone who will be willing to lend a shoulder or input for support.

I felt bad for myself for a long time. I think we feel bad for ourselves for far too long. We tend to use bipolar as a crutch. Now, don't get me wrong: bipolar was one hell of a reason to get out of plans. I use that shit to this day. I remember I'd say, "You don't understand! I'm bipolar!" There was a long time where I felt so bad for myself and wondered why so many unfair things had happened to me. *Why do I have to take medicine to be okay? Why did I go through this? Why why why? Why me?* It's okay and normal to feel that way *for a time.* But not for a *long* time.

Keep that mentality; it's okay for a minute. But you need to move on at some point and start to climb out of this hole.

I started exercising again. I started trying to do things to rebuild who I was before, and what that meant for me was going to the gym. It always made me feel good. Hanging out with friends always made me feel good, but I had to take baby steps. I couldn't just fall in with twenty friends. It was just Nick and Krystina, baby steps. I couldn't just go to the gym all the time and be totally happy, but I would say to myself, *Phylecia, you've got to get to the gym a couple times this week. Do one small thing a day to go in the right direction.*

What changed it all: I woke up one day, and maybe I had had a conversation with my dad. I don't know what it was. But I swear to God, it was like a switch went off, like my friend mentioned in her passage. There was a long time where I was angry and had pity for myself. Then, a thought came over me. *Wait a second, there are so many people who have disorders. Some people can't go take a walk by themselves. Some people have suffered major loss in their lives. It's not "Why me?" It's "Why the fuck NOT me?"*

Why would I be any different from any other human who has suffered from trauma, has been diagnosed with a disorder, has an ailment, or must take medications to "be okay"?

Let's find the solution.

"Why not me?" That was the shift.

I was coming back.

I'll be damned.

I was finally letting go of the endless cycle of bullshit and pity. The change was the mindset shift. I finally asked the right question: *Why NOT me?*

That attitude opened the doors. Suddenly, I could see a light shining at the end of the tunnel. *Hell, there's a solution for this. I don't have to stay here and pity piss-poor me.*

It seems like a small shift, but it was huge. This was the beginning of my comeback season.

Have you ever seen those Japanese bowls that have been broken and then put back together? They have cool gold plates and all kinds of cool designs on them where the cracks have been joined. Because they've been put back together, they look way more interesting. I'd seen those before, so I looked up the history online. The exact origins are unknown, but apparently there was someone who fixed a bowl that had been broken at some point, and then the practice of *intentionally* joining tea bowls with powdered gold became widespread in Japan in the sixteenth century.

Let's say before your episode you were a navy blue, regular Joe bowl. Nothing too great about it, but nothing broken about it. It worked fine. Well, that bowl crashed into one thousand pieces. If you want to save that bowl, you're gonna have to glue that shit back together. But what if you did it the Japanese way, gluing it back together with all those cool gold pieces?

That looks way more interesting. It's way stronger than it ever was before.

Write down right now: Who is your support? Who do *you* support? What is your daily routine, your daily check-in? What books can you read to get help? Who can you listen to to receive real feedback?

What are your own triggers and onsets for mania? For depression? Now, what the hell are you going to do if in five minutes a wave of depression comes on? What about mania? You need to know this right now, today—not tomorrow.

Once you have these pieces in place, you become the boss. Bipolar is just a part of your game; it's not the entire picture. It will sometimes throw a wrench in your plans, but you take that wrench and launch it the fuck out.

Once you have this foundation nailed down and understand what these components mean to you, the sunshine will begin to appear, and it will stay for longer stretches of time.

There is no reason to use this disorder as an excuse for bad behavior or for disassociating from life and responsibilities long-term.

Remember, for a *time*, those struggles are normal. But after six months (if not sooner), you need to start getting your game face on.

Now we're entering the world of gluing our lives and ourselves back together bit by bit. You should be becoming stable. You should now have a routine and plans, starting each day prepared and ready.

I want you now to start taking baby steps forward. My therapist said something to me years ago that is now a tagline:

KEEP TRUDGING FORWARD.

That's it. That's all we're doing right now. Baby-step the shit out of life, until things get easier, and you can become more advanced.

You're going to take a step toward your next pivotal moment. What makes you laugh? What makes you feel *good* about yourself?

Right here, this is still all about you and your comeback season.

Your entire life does not have to be based on "I'm bipolar so I can't XYZ." F* that mess. You can do all the things, and you don't have to be manic while you're at it.

You need not live in fear of "what if" you feel bad again; you will. It comes with the territory, so get over that fear and instead focus on what to do next—because you're working on your own strategy to come out of it.

Today, I am totally content just to *be*. I don't have to live up to a certain standard. I don't have to worry about what other people think. I am not just the entertainment. There are times when I love to be the center of attention, but I don't have to be. I don't feel the need to make *sure* I'm the center of attention. I don't feel that pressure anymore.

What a relief.

One more quickie story for ya.

My nephew broke his arm last year. It damn near snapped like a twig. He was seven years old, jumped off a swing, and fell wrong. Both bones between the wrist and elbow of his little arm were broken. The X-ray was rough, I'll tell ya.

The doctor told us, and I quote: "Since we have to fuse that part of his arm back together on purpose, that part of his arm that is broken in half is going to be stronger than it was before."

Let me reiterate; **it is going to be stronger than it was before it was broken**.

I don't know if the same is physically true for adult bones as it is for kids, but the metaphor still holds: the broken part that will heal stronger than ever is *you*. Since you've got to repair your life, with purpose and intention, you will come back stronger than you ever were before. You are stronger than you ever *had* to be before. You will become untouchable. You have tools in your toolbox that you never needed before. Be the broken arm that comes back stronger.

That's what learning how to breathe again is all about.

Takeaways

Absorb the fact that you can learn how to breathe again and make a comeback.

Life cannot be all about you all the time; find someone else to help.

Be like my nephew's broken arm: come back stronger than you've ever been before.

Let's get to work.

Chapter 10
Confidence, Independence, and Joy

"Strength and growth come only through continuous effort and struggle."

—Napoleon Hill

You must be stable to enter this next stage.

Over the course of your life, these stages will become more advanced. There will be times in your life when you'll feel independent because you were able to get coffee by yourself. Then there will be times when you buy a home, upgrade to a nicer apartment, break up with the idiot, or travel on your own. Things get better and better, but for right now, let's talk about how you begin to gain your confidence and worth back.

For me, confidence was everything. I was so confident in high school, that I was bullied but still came out on top. I'm talking intense bullying too. This kid told me things like, "You need to keep going to the tanning bed, so you get skin cancer and die." He screamed at me in class, had a "bodyguard" intimidate me outside of the classroom, and talked mad shit within earshot. He wrote pages and pages on social media about how big my nose was, saying I looked like Toucan Sam—which I then got a shirt of and set as my profile picture on Facebook, just to show I didn't give a shit. He called me an Oompa Loompa and said I was going to be a server like my mom for the rest of my life because I couldn't get into a university. (I got accepted to University of Kentucky and was moving to Utah for school, LOL.)

This dude didn't faze me at all. When people would tell me what he said, I was like, "I have no idea why this is important," and went about my business. When the ole girl stood outside my classroom to act like she was going to jump me, I walked straight past her with my shoulders back and head held high.

I tell you this story because confidence is *everything.* Not only will it set you apart, it will also protect you. When you walk tall and know who you are, people naturally don't fuck with you. If you are a sheep and look like one, people take advantage. If you are bullied and don't have the right head on your shoulders, shit can go sideways.

That's why gaining your confidence and self-esteem back is paramount to your entire life's trajectory.

The reason I also talk about confidence, independence, and joy is because those three things go hand in hand. If you feel independent, that brings confidence. With those two in place, you most likely have joy somewhere or will find it soon.

You must work on one of these three, whichever comes first for you—in that way, life blooms.

But by this stage of the Bipolar Life Cycle, you should not be in survival mode anymore. Once I started branching out, I gained independence and confidence by getting my office job. I was so happy to be able to drive to the office, get my coffee, go to my cubicle, and work.

When I got my own apartment again in 2014, it was about two hundred square feet. I could pivot and be in my living room, bedroom, office, and kitchen all at once. Who knew you could be in four places at one time?! Still, it was a great feeling. I was on my own again. I felt totally content spending time by myself, laughing at comedy shows, making videos, dubbing over movies I loved, having fifty dollars to spend at the grocery store every two weeks, and getting dog food, peanut butter, bread, and carrots. It was life.

But what did this bring? I didn't know it at the time at all, but because I was able to take care of these responsibilities, I felt independent again. That gave me self-esteem, which brought joy. I didn't have a weight on my shoulders anymore, though I knew it would periodically come and go for the rest of my life.

I was so grateful not to be in the state I'd experienced years before. I could not believe I was making other people laugh again. I could not believe I could sit on my couch and be at peace—no racing thoughts, no anxiety, no terrible depression telling me I was a loser.

I had joy in myself because I knew I could laugh again—I was free.

I'll be damned.

Things started getting better and better, and then I experienced another pivotal moment: my nephew, Malikai, was born in June 2015. You'll hear more about him later, but when he came around, I was so happy that I could be who I needed to be for him and my sister.

I upgraded to a nicer apartment in 2016. By this time, I had been going out again and hanging out with all kinds of friends. I was having a damn ball.

In this stage of my life, my focus was on coming back socially and having an easy, stable job. I didn't want to juggle. I had quality time with my nephew, family, and friends.

I did not consciously know what I was doing at the time. I was not thinking to myself, *Step 1: Map out plan; Step 2: Solutions; Step 3: Learn to breathe again; Step 4: Find confidence, independence, and joy; Step 5: Focus on social aspects.*

No, I was just ready, and I took life step by step. When I was ready to get a better job, I got one. When I was ready to move out, I did. When I had the ability to start working out and eating healthier, that's where my focus went.

I felt like myself again. The blonde, funny chick who makes dumb jokes and has a ballin'-ass time—she was here and back at it.

Be happy for the small steps forward.

Since I had missed out on ages twenty-one to twenty-five, when I came back, people had already done the early-twenties thing. I was held back. I was ready to go *wild*, and I sure did. I dated some idiots, but ya live, ya learn.

When I upgraded to my new apartment, I also upgraded my car. That's right: a Jeep Wrangler hardtop. I had arrived. I was so proud of my apartment and my car. People would ask, "What's your dream car?"

My response? "Shit, I'm living the dream, baby—this is it."

My apartment was expensive to some, but to me, it was everything. I was happy to pay. It was clean, it was mine, and I had a beautiful yard for my dog. I had worked at home since about 2015, and I loved my life. It was easy, no pressure at all. I did not want any other stress in my life. I'd been stressed and riddled with anxiety, worry, and doubt for years. I wanted to live easy and free. That's exactly what I did.

Some of this sounds materialistic, but the point is, I was capable of living on my own again and was able to start loving the life I lived. You will too.

I didn't care about what I wanted to "do for the rest of my life." I was perfectly content and happy. But I also knew that I was bipolar. I did not get cocky. I always took my meds and stayed on the path of mental health and stability. You must get to that even-keeled maintenance phase to start living your real life. Being bipolar does not define you.

I have lived through it. I have been there, done that—bought the T-shirt and took that shit straight back.

This diagnosis is totally manageable, if you do the work.

As you gain confidence, independence, and joy again, things just go up from there.

Now listen, of course life happens. Of course, you are still bipolar, and trauma can happen—but you are beginning to have building blocks. Tools. Solutions. A foundation.

With these in place, we come back quicker and easier.

Once things get easy, it's time for a new challenge, a new idea, a new job, a new hobby. You're ready to advance and develop. It's time to read a book, time to listen to someone who's awesome and where you want to be.

I also don't compare myself to *anyone*, good or bad. Your path is *yours* and yours only. Your battle is between you and you. No one else.

I sometimes wish I were farther down the road but enjoy the ride. Be happy you're not down in the dumps. Be happy you got through your trauma.

Be happy—or get the fuck out.

Go to your best day. What are you doing? What are you wearing? Who are you with? What type of music are you listening to? Go there and get that clarity back. Then start with a "How do I achieve that?" action plan to make your current life better.

One. Step. At. A. Time.

Confidence: What do you want to feel confident in—i.e., where do you find worth, self-esteem, and value? Whatever it is, do the damn thing. What makes you feel *good* about yourself?

Independence: What areas do you want independence in? Do you want to pay your own car insurance? Do you want to own your own home or live by yourself? Do you want to travel? The goal can be small first; over time, it will grow.

Joy: What brings you joy? What makes you laugh? What brings peace and warmth to your heart? Is it doing good for others, being of service? You must know this stuff to learn to be in love with being alive.

Once you have these pieces in place, dear God, you can only go up from there—because you are beginning to know who you are and what you enjoy, or what you could enjoy. It doesn't matter what other people are doing. Do you.

As long as it's safe, happy, and healthy, rock on.

Takeaways

Becoming independent and confident again represents a huge milestone. After you get stable, ask yourself: *What can bring me independence? Where can I find worth in myself again?* Regaining self-esteem is everything, as it will bring joy.

You see, it's all a cycle. Things will get better over time. At some points in your life, you could be independent in that you are able to go home and feel totally content by yourself. At others, it could look like being able to travel alone. It means different things for different people, but what we're all building back is our self-worth, self-esteem, and sense of value.

Chapter 11
Belief System

Searching: Mormon, to Be or Not to Be?

Clarifying your belief system is important to the process of gaining control. We'll always be searching to some extent, but the way we do so changes over the course of our lives and our recovery.

I think your belief system, your morals, and what you stand for are a huge piece of your foundation. If you don't stand for something, you'll fall for anything. What happens when the loss of a loved one comes? What are you going to do? Who will you turn to?

When I got out of the hospital, I experienced the part of depression that involves blame and guilt. I blamed myself because I wasn't on the straight and narrow, and God only knows what can happen. I thought I deserved this. I decided I should start going to church again and clean up my life.

You see, I was raised Mormon. When you're Mormon, you're taught to believe that you should be living valiantly, and if you're not on the straight and narrow, bad things happen.

Before my manic episode, let's just say I wasn't on the straight and narrow.

I started to blame myself for what seemed like the consequences. I felt ashamed. I thought, *Well, this is why. You are being punished for knowing what's right, knowing what the "true church" believes, and choosing to do otherwise.*

It seemed like God didn't care about me anymore. Maybe he did because I was a child of God, but because I wasn't active in the church and living right, the spirit was no longer with me. I believed that's why things had gone off the rails.

I began going back to church. I believed that if I got back on the path, things would begin to change. I believed that if I lived in the way I had in high school, my spark would come back.

I remember having a conversation (more like a confession) with one member of the bishopric— sort of like a "preacher's assistant," but we had bishops instead of preachers. I told him what had happened and how I was living before. I remember saying, "I know why I don't have the light shining in me anymore. It's because I wasn't living right. I haven't been active or living in the way I know I was raised to."

He said, "I'm happy you see that." In other words, he agreed that part of the reason this episode had happened, or part of the reason I felt so shitty, was because I wasn't living in the manner the church taught. Once again, someone in power figuratively slapped me in the face, like my psychiatrist had years before.

That is what I would come to know as bullshit later.

But at this time, I accepted it. I thought, *Yep, that's part of the reason. I am to blame for this.*

I do want to preface this as well: I will not slay this church. This church was why I was who I was growing up. I had pride in being Mormon. I still have amazing friends who are Mormon. There are so many good people. There are so many great belief systems the church has, including some I still believe now. I have respect for this religion.

What didn't happen was this: maybe a year into being active in the church again, I didn't feel any closer to God or spirituality. I wasn't connected to it. I wasn't drinking or smoking weed. I was close to my parents, trying to do the right thing—but somehow, I began doubting the church.

Then something happened.

A friend who was a member of the church came out as homosexual. I won't say his name here as it's not my place, but he is proud of who he is, and so am I. I'll call him Ted (because I love the show *Ted Lasso*).

He was a guy whom members of the church described as "an angel sent straight from heaven."

Ted was gay, and my dad always knew. When Ted was about fourteen years old, my dad met him and knew right off the bat that he was gay. It just was a fact; he also knew that when Ted came out, he was going to have one helluva problem in the church.

I didn't take it too seriously. If Ted was gay, cool; if not, cool. I went on about my business. I loved Ted. He was so warm to everyone he met. I remember one time it was Valentine's Day, and I was babysitting for a couple at church. Ted came over and brought me a rose and Olive Garden takeout and sat with me on Valentine's Day. He knew I was single and that I was also babysitting. That's the heart this dude had. Who even does that at age fourteen?

Then a moment changed my life: we learned that Ted would be accepted in the church only if he "never acted on his feelings or physical attraction to men."

That solidified my thoughts toward the church. I then started to believe that maybe this church wasn't so perfect after all.

I don't know what you believe, but I don't believe that being gay is a choice. It is part of who you are as a person. Some people were never meant to be married to the opposite sex. We knew Ted was gay early on. Who cares? He was and is one of the kindest people I had ever known. How can he be wrong?

I then started doing some research on the Mormon church and slowly began my exit. I couldn't relate to the church anymore. At the core, being a Mormon wasn't who I wanted to be.

I think there is a time in many people's lives when we start questioning and searching.

When I started really questioning the church, this is what dawned on me that I couldn't ignore: most people I knew weren't Mormon, yet they had beautiful lives. They were good people. My best friend Darian was living with her now-husband, who was her boyfriend of ten years. She lived in Florida at the time and was living her best life. She had a light in her eyes. She wasn't Mormon, so how did she have a light and shine?

I also began to think, *Wait a second. I didn't do anything worse than the next guy to make me "fall into a bipolar episode." I wasn't being punished. That's horse shit. It just happened.* I had a chemical imbalance in my brain, and it was my problem to solve.

I began developing my own belief system. I believe in God, a higher power, or the universe.

I believe that your God is where you feel at peace and happy. My dad's God is nature. My dad's God is his family, music, and laughter. Some people's God is seeing a butterfly and hearing the birds chirp on a sunny day. Some people's God is a religious one. My God and my belief system are now spiritual. I still pray daily, and I believe that going to church is good for the soul. I think kids love church because they feel good while they're there.

I didn't *not* believe in something before, but to me, what happened in my next story made it undeniable that there is something bigger than me out there.

In 2019, I had my life back. I had my friends, and my dog Smokey lived with me. I had a beautiful backyard that I enjoyed every day.

This one day, I was waiting for one of my girlfriends to come over, and I was sitting out on my little porch. I had the water jug I brought back from Key West from Darian's wedding a year prior. I was smoking a Black & Mild. It was a gorgeous, sunny fall day in Kentucky. Smokey was lying beside me, enjoying being outside with his person. I had an Alexa on. The song "Crash" by Dave Matthews started playing. This song had meaning because when I was little, my dad used to play it, and it also became a song my friend Jon and I listened to all the time. We love Dave Matthews Band. It was a moment in time I will never forget.

The air was breathing just right. The birds were singing. I saw the trees waving back to me.

The perfect song came on. First, I got the chills. Then I started crying. These weren't tears of sorrow—they were the truest tears of gratitude I had ever shed.

I believe in that moment, God was right next to me.

Writing about this experience brought me to tears again. I began to think of all the tough experiences of my past—and all the time when I believed I could never feel this way again. Yet there I was, so happy, so content, so at ease and thankful for what my life had become. For years, just feeling good one moment at a time was something I'd considered impossible. I reveled in that moment. I didn't want it to end. I was inside that moment—the moment I believe new moms feel when they are with their babies the first time, those quiet, peaceful, thankful places that sometimes seem few and far between.

In that moment, I knew who my God was—moments like this. From that day on, I've lived inside each moment like that one. I stop to smell the coffee, to hear the birds sing, to look at my beautiful nephew's smile and think of his pure heart. I think about my parents and my sister. I think about my friends and the love we have for each other.

Eight years before, I couldn't think this way. I couldn't think of good times from the past. But at that moment, I believed you don't have to be Mormon to feel the spirit. If that wasn't the spirit or feeling something greater than me—I don't know what is.

Sometimes, when you're living right, shit happens right. When you're in tune with yourself and the beautiful world around you, those moments happen. Life can be hard, and there's ugliness in the world—but when those moments happen, stop. Notice them. Be grateful.

Live in the good moments for as long as you can and remember them on the hard days.

I found my own belief system.

I'll be damned.

Takeaways

When you begin to feel the need to search in your life, scratch that itch. (Just watch out for cults.) I needed to find my own belief system, which offered a new level of stability and answers. If you don't stand for something, you'll fall for anything.

Chapter 12
Bringing Back Gratitude

"When asked if my cup is half full or half empty, my only response is that I am thankful I have a cup."

—Sam Lefkowitz

I found gratitude three or four years after being diagnosed. It tends to come on its own in time. You want to find it as quickly as possible, but remember your own process comes first.

Gratitude is a part of this process that will be huge for your own well-being. We're not in fight-or-flight mode, and we're not in survival mode—we are now understanding what life is about.

So what is gratitude? Many sources define it as the quality of being thankful, ready to show appreciation, and willing to return kindness.

The turning point for me was feeling grateful for my diagnosis.

If it weren't for being bipolar, I wouldn't have had to understand how to be mentally healthy. The challenge showed me even if I'm dealt a bad hand, I can find tools. Every day is a great day to be alive, because I now know this is beatable.

I never would have known what it's like to fall and rise back up. I never would have known struggle and anguish and, as a result, never would have found true happiness.

When you struggle, when you sink so low and come back up, you begin to be grateful for things you never would have noticed before.

Let's talk about how to start finding true happiness in your own life.

Pivotal moment: When I thanked God that I was diagnosed early on enough to be present for my sister when my nephew came, that was it. More doors opened.

My sister and I were not the best of friends in 2014. She came to me with some news—she was pregnant. I knew I was going to be instrumental in helping her raise this kid. She needed help. She was young, and we are now co-parents in Malikai's life. If I had not been stable and "back" to Phylecia by this time, I never would have been able to show up like I did for her and for him.

He would have not had the support and love that I know I can give. Ashley wouldn't have had the support she needed in the care of her son. She is grateful for the help, yes, but *I* am also so grateful I had the ability to do that for her. If this had been five years prior, I would have been off the rails and dissociated completely.

I realized this: *Wait a second, if it was inevitable that I was bipolar and I was going to have a manic episode at some point—how thankful am I that this thing manifested in time for me to get my shit together before my nephew was born?!*

If that's not a revelation, I don't know what is. I was grateful for the divine timing. The universe, God, or whoever is out there knew something: *This girl is going to have a real responsibility here in a few years. This thing needs to manifest so that she can rip the band-aid off, work on healing, and come back in time to be ready.*

That's exactly how I see it. That's being in tune with your star player (as Katt Williams would say).

When I look into my nephew's eyes, I know I was meant to be one of his parents. He is the pure joy of my life, along with his little sister Brielle who came along last year. It has been my privilege to help bring him up, and I will care for him until I die. I am who I am, but I know I was meant to coach him and teach him about safety, confidence, independence, and his own joy.

He is *one* of my purposes, which we will get into in part IV. But again, if I hadn't been diagnosed until even a few years later than I was, there is no way I could have done what I did or have been who I needed to be for Malikai and Ashley at that time.

The stars aligned for me in 2010, when I had my episode. Maybe it's a good thing that I smoked a lot of weed, because it helped the mania manifest quickly and dramatically—just in time to be diagnosed and on the road to recovery by 2014.

That sense of optimism, abundance, and gratitude is how we need to look at life. Once you can see the forest for the trees, your mindset will shift every time.

One practice that will help put you on this path and maintain the mindset is daily gratitude. Author, amazing podcaster, speaker, businesswoman, and my personal favorite, Rachel Hollis, talks a lot about gratitude and keeping a daily journal. I love the idea of looking for gratitude in our everyday lives, because it helps us live with a glass-half-full mindset. On the other hand, if we go into every day looking at the negative, how we spilled our coffee, how we were late, and so on, we live with the glass half-empty. If you change your perspective, it's wild what you can really see.

Because of our struggles, bipolar people can find gratitude and be happy in ways others can't.

If you are bipolar, or have been down a tough road, the fact that you made it here means you survived. If you have been in a hole and come out of it, you can be grateful for even the most mundane of days!

Let me explain. People who have not suffered from terrible, clinical depression could be asked about their day and say, "Eh, just another day at the office."

But for bipolar person, *just another day at the office? Shit, I'm happy as hell this was just another day at the office! That means I freakin' made it without losing my shit. I made it and worked all day with no cloud of depression over me. It's a great day to be alive!*

We can see beauty in ways others can't. That's something to be hella grateful for.

That's how we can see the world. To us, we've been so low that we *longed* for a normal day. We longed for a day when we just didn't feel shitty. We wanted so badly to be able to go to work and feel *fine*, normal, centered.

We longed for "just another day at the office."

When you get there, oh my Lord, what a great feeling. I used to wake up and feel a weight on me. It was so hard to do normal tasks that I thought I'd never be myself again. I felt a gray cloud over me, and it was suffocating.

Finally, I got out from under that cloud and recognized the days when I didn't feel that way. For each one of those, I am so grateful. And the days that are even better, when something especially good happens, I am out of this world excited (which is where hypomania can come in that we must watch for).

On New Year's Day 2024, I spent the day at my parents' house, sitting on the couch with my nephew, watching movies in our pajamas. There was a time when trying to sit down made me so uncomfortable—with myself, with my brain activity, with the feeling of my heart pounding. There was no peace, no relaxation at all.

But on New Year's this past year? None of that. I was so happy to be there, to feel comfortable with who I am. My heart wasn't pounding, and my hands weren't shaking. I was there and happy, content. I stopped what we were doing and said, "We need to remember days like this."

Hold on to those good times for as long as you can, and then write about them. Remember them on the bad days.

I am famous for being with my friends or family and stopping an entire night or event to say, "These are the good ole days—we need to remember this moment."

It's important to live with intention but also be mindful of the fact that you aren't in a state of madness or anxiety. Right now, as I'm writing this, I am free. Nothing fantastic has happened today, but damn, I'm not depressed, and that's a great day either way.

When you practice being grateful and living inside the good moments, then when the bad moments happen, you can hop out of them quicker.

Our job is to understand that the more gratitude we have for the good, the more frequently we will find it.

When I was on my swim team and we'd have a long, grueling workout, I'd keep looking at the clock and saying, "Nothing lasts, nothing lasts." That's what kept me going until that hand reached the 5:30 p.m. mark.

In a way, that sounds negative: nothing lasts. But of course, the great days aren't going to be every single day, and neither are the bad days. There's power in knowing that.

When you feel the depression coming on, you have to tell yourself, *Nothing lasts*, and work on getting out of it.

Be thankful you can identify it, respect it, and move on.

Be thankful for "just another day at the office."

Be thankful for the sole fact that you survived thus far and you're working on becoming a better version of yourself.

Be thankful that you can be thankful for the mundane and ordinary. No news is good news sometimes, right?

Be thankful you made it to today, to reading this book. Many others didn't. Now, let's go find your magic.

Takeaways

Gratitude and seeing the beauty in life are everything. Be a glass-half-full kinda guy.

Because of our struggles, we can be grateful for things that others take for granted.

Part IV
Thriving

Before entering our final part, "Thriving," read through my journal entries. You can clearly see how my mindset and life changed in thirteen years. In Part I, I was sad and felt alone. Here, I am excited about my life and what's to come, updating instead of longing for happiness. You will get there too!

Today Carroll & my mom are out of town & Poppa's at work so its just me & mal chillin. we should be outside but I was tired after work so here we are. mal stayed home from camp today & I told him no TV - Be creative. when I was done w/ work the house was a mess but hey - he was creative. he better own his own Biz one day. we've been told he has touch of Adhd But when he's interested in something, all attn is on it. he ♡s learning what words mean & he's so inquisitive abt life. loves working on stuff w/ Poppa Built swing set, bed etc - loves ninja stuff, just started tackle football. he ♡s it but worn out. he's gotta get whipped into shape. he broke his arm a few months ago when he jumped off a swing - so he's been chillin for awhile - Ashley had another Baby! She came on may 5th? 2023 or 1st?

her name is Brielle Rae - she's a doll
looks so much like Terrell but is so
pretty. mal is a great big brother -
when Ash in hospital mal couldn't wait
to come. wherever Brielle was, he was
he could have stayed all 3 days.
Ash had c section - she's doing really
well. she's an anxiety mess & in
therapy. you can tell she's cut out
for it & has the mom thing nailed
down.
on the
for th
been d
4 wks.
my mom doing great. broke back when
she went sledding w/ mal in Dec.
mal stayed right next 2 her the whole
time. she's still active & we try to
tell her to be careful! she works
at lowes for 4-5 hr shifts - wish
she could retire.

I've always known I'm meant for something Big & never knew what always wanted 2 be on stage, never knew how - this is it! Allie has been helping, she's amazing she helped w/ content & video posting, baby steps, & logo & course subjects I never would have known where to start. I've been doing 1/2 vids/wk since January I'm on youtube, FB & IG. trying 2 Build following - got my associates last yr & started writing my Book. have part 1 & 2 Done (roughly) & tomorrow going to Lexington for my "writing retreat" to finish part 3 - this journal helped write part 2 - also want to finish courses so maybe I can make recurring rev - Big dream is to have podcast, group coaching, FB group - Biggest dream - travel & Do speaking events (be on stage) Shane's mom said when I left for Utah "you're going 2 do something Big" & That always stayed w/me

I got to see Dahan "3 times in 1 semester"!! we saw Johnny Depp in real life!! we came to the palace - we went to the stage & were crying w/ excitement - It was so cool! seeing ~~Johnny~~ in real life?? he was playing in a band quotes - "if someone tells us to back up we will fuckin fight"
we waited outside 2 see his tour bus leave + ppl w/ us helped me take off my boots lol - we were 1st row of ppl + made friends w/ the cute security gaurds so they let us stay up there w/ them while telling everyone to "Backup" a little 8 yr old was trying to inch up & I said "you better get that kid - I will stomp an 8yr old" hahaha - we saw Johnny! he doesnt know this - But he literally saw us, he made total eye contact w/ us & it was so cool - Dare was Blowing kisses & ~~I~~ yours truly just pointed at him & nodded lol like yaas youre the shit

lets see what else - last year in march of 2022 I went on solo trip to chicago + michigan - It was amazing - you know I went for a 3 week solo trip up north I hope right? that was in 2018, nyc, cape cod, maine niagara - in 2021 I took parents + mae on that same trip condensed - when I was in michigan back to 3/2022 it was still winter there. was driving up in mountains, had bear spray [redacted] w/me - thank god b/c my ass got stuck! car got stuck in snow w/out a soul or service in sight. had to walk a mile just to get service 2 get pulled out. It was a fantastic time I was prepared + cautious but shit it brings character - [redacted] goes "omg did that ruin your trip??" - maybe wand for a wack like her

for me - it only made it more interesting
I ♡ed it & had a great story to tell

Idk man life is great - I've
gained way too much weight
that's always on my mind so
I've gotta buckle down & look &
Phyl good - see what I did there?
Wall & I have a great time - he's
currently making another huge
mess w/ a glue gun but jacket
we'll clean it up he's such a
good kid. we love the matilda
song "all the way" & "Days like this"
by van morrison - makes me
cry to listen 2 them w/ him
I ♡ seeing just sing to a song.
also free falling reminds me of
my mom - she's a good girl,
loves her momma, ♡ horses &
her bf too, she's a good girl
crazy 'bout elvis, ♡s jesus &
America too - something like
that - so other than needing
lose 50 lbs - life is good - wish me
luck on buying this land!
♡ Phyl

Chapter 13
Finding Your Magic

Let's Fall in Love with Being Alive

"We're living life anyway. The time is going to pass either way. We might as well chip away at our dreams in the meantime."

—Olivia McDaniel, entrepreneur
and my personal big-picture,
get-your-shit-together friend

I inserted those journal entries before this part of the book because it's vital that you see the difference between the person who wrote the journal entries from 2010 at the beginning of the book and the person who wrote the ones in 2022. Technically I'm the same person, but I've also progressed and become totally different.

Thriving really means we are becoming successful in our bipolar journey. We will never be "cured," and we will never be completely done. It's like doing laundry or staying sober. Laundry is never complete. It may be done for the day—but we know it's inevitable that we will have to wash, dry, and fold the clothes all over again. We know ups and downs are inevitable. But we can now continue our growth.

At this stage, we are in love with being alive or trying to be. We enjoy our lives, and we can live authentically as ourselves. With those pieces in place, we can move on to even bigger things. We can continue to grow by taking on a new adventure, a new challenge, a new idea, a dream we've always had. We have the right to enjoy the moment, and we have the focus to grow. We are not stunted or stuck. We can see even more light because we are not constantly worried about our disorder or what could happen. We know what could happen, and we've got a plan for its ass.

Know you are not alone. You continue your path, keep your integrity, and stand for something. Follow these steps and go back to them if you believe you're flailing again.

Write down your plans, tools, tactics, and strategies. Write down what brings you purpose, confidence, independence, and joy. Write down your favorite quotes and song lyrics. Read the good books and listen to the right people. Get your house in order (figuratively and literally). If you have a dream, it can be achieved—take strides in that direction. Manage your disorder early on so that you can move on more quickly.

When you engage in these practices and this preparation, you don't have to live in a state of worry and doubt. You accept and move on. You begin to live and love.

I may swerve, take a couple U-turns, and need to get back on track occasionally—but I know I'm at least on the right path. We're on our way.

At this stage, start with these questions:

- Who do you want to be for the rest of your life?
- What do you want to bring to the table that is life?
- What is your equivalent of the Super Bowl?

Now that we have the foundation in place, we want to *thrive*. Life is not all about bipolar. Bipolar is something that happened—we will always need to respect its power and stay committed to our mental health—but now we are reentering the world.

Pivotal Moment: The Solo Road Trip, 2018 —Personal Development

There will be times in your life when the ability to ask different questions will come. In 2018, I started searching again.

Eight years prior to this, there had been no wondering. I hadn't asked, "What have I always wanted to do?" I was only surviving. But now that I had my life back together, I was able to see through my own bullshit and ask different questions. You will get here.

I asked myself, *what is something I've always wanted to do?* I thought, *Man, I have always wanted to travel by myself. How freakin' cool would that be? Just take a road trip and be on my own and do what I want, when I want.*

During this same exact time, my BFF Darian sent me some books, including *You Are a Badass* by Jen Sincero. In that book, she says something like "take the trip—just do it." Those words solidified my decision: I was going. (*Side note*: What a God thing or universe thing to have a book say exactly what I needed to hear!)

I proceeded to book a three-week-long solo road trip northeast.

My first stop? New York City. I spent three days in the city (safe and back to my hotel by 6:00 p.m. every day). I was able to gallivant and see many things! It was so much fun. I saw someone wearing a hat from Keeneland (a racetrack in Kentucky) the same day I had a Keeneland shirt on among hundreds of people in line, and we chatted. It turned out they lived right down the street from where I lived in Kentucky!

There was comfort in knowing there were familiar people around in a big city like New York. I saw *The Lion King* on Broadway and felt a bit sad because of all the families, but guess who I sat between? Two other single women who were traveling by themselves. It was the most amazing thing. I got to go through the 9/11 Memorial, which was super important to me, and I went on a ferry around Manhattan to see Lady Liberty.

To me, New York was a metaphor. It was somewhere I'd always wanted to go, and there's something patriotic about that city. I took great pride in being there. I also kept myself open to the experience, and by doing so, I was able to find many wonderful people around me.

I made my way up to Cape Cod. I had always wanted to go there ever since I saw the movie *Splash* as a kid with Tom Hanks. It was gorgeous. The one time I did feel a bit sad and alone was in Cape Cod, when I had had a long day and missed my family. But I knew what to do: I Face Timed Malikai and said family prayers with everyone, and then off I went.

From there, I went to Maine and Niagara Falls to finish the trip. I met so many amazing people, but more than that? I was completely happy and at peace—something that, years before, I'd thought would never happen again.

I had this shit scheduled down to the minute so I could do as much as possible, while also enjoying the beauty and not knowing what day it was.

My sister reminded me to put this section in the book as this was *The* Comeback. She said it still makes her emotional to this day because there was a time when I couldn't leave my mom's side. I never wanted to be alone. She said, "When you booked that trip and left, I knew you had completely made it back, and I was so happy for you. You have to include that in your book."

As you gain more confidence and independence in your life, you'll then have the means to ask the next question. My question in 2018 was "What have I always wanted to do?" The answer was to travel solo. And so, I went.

During the trip, nothing life-changing happened; the big transformation came after the trip. It was knowing I had done something I had always wanted to do and loved every single second of it. I took great pride in my solo road trip and still do. I have taken other trips now too, but that was the beginning.

It changed my trajectory on so many different levels. It opened the doors to thinking bigger for my life.

If I did that, what else could I do?

Pivotal Moment: The Sales Gig, 2021 —Professional Development and Choosing My Destiny

A couple years later, the questions changed again. I was working at the office job I told you about before. I had been working there since 2014. It was the answer for a time, but then it got too easy.

I was not concerned with who I wanted to be or what I was meant to do, because I wasn't there yet. I was solely focused on learning what I loved, traveling, taking care of the people I loved, and fulfilling a need in being a parent and guardian to my nephew. When I was back socially, I loved my life again.

But I remember talking to my therapist and saying, "I know I'm meant to do something, but I just don't know what it is. It's not taking care of my nephew. It's not traveling."

And she was like, "Yeah, no, that's not it."

I went back to school to finish my associate's degree. I only needed five classes, So I thought, *Okay, I'll finish my associate's, and maybe I'll go back to school to get my license to be a therapist. I love my therapist; she's awesome. I love talking to people and helping. Maybe that's it.*

I wondered now, *what am I supposed to do?* It was time for a new challenge. Who was I meant to be now that I had my life back in order?

Finally, when the dust settled and I found myself only able to pay my bills and live paycheck to paycheck, this thought came to me: *I am wasting my only real talent. It's talking to people. What's that mean? What can I do with that?* I thought at the time it was becoming a therapist.

That wasn't it.

A lot of this is really knowing who to take advice from and who not to take advice from.

I reached out to my friend Allie. She owns her own business, and I knew she knew me and would have great insight. She said, "Phylecia, your dream is not to be a therapist. You don't want to sit in a room all day and talk to people. You have a story, and it's meant to be shared. You need to be a bipolar success coach. You need to write a book."

I rolled my eyes and laughed. She was the entrepreneur, not me. I thought I needed to go to school to get a degree and just have a career. But the longer I sat with it, the more the idea resonated with me. Allie gave me what I needed: clarity.

Clarity is everything. I thought, *Wait a second, yeah, I don't want to just sit in an office all day and talk to people about their problems. That's not it.*

When I wrapped my mind around the fact that she could be onto something about me writing a book, I wondered if I was going a little manic again.

That stopped me in my tracks. Was it mania? Was I going crazy again?

I told Allie, and she said, "Phylecia, you are not manic. This is not delusional. You're not talking to the TV. You are dreaming. You are trying to find out what *you* love and what you really want to do. Entrepreneurs get excited about that, and they *do* things. They find the path. They all are a little ADHD and high-energy; they have to be."

The point is: I wasn't manic. In fact, I had found the clarity I needed.

Then it went further. When I got on this idea, the wheels started turning. I said, "Okay, if I wrote a book, what would that look like? I can't just make money doing that, and it's not my life's dream to be a coach—although that's amazing and a perfect way to spend my time and make money doing something I love." I realized I could share my story and help other people in a way that I wasn't helped. I was onto something.

Then it went further. I asked myself, *What lights my fire? What ignites my passion?* It's the dream I've always had of being on stage.

But I'm not a comedian, I can't sing, and I'm not a Broadway actor. I found it: I'm supposed to be a speaker. There it is—like a magician revealing the rabbit in the hat.

My entire life, I've loved being on stage. I love entertaining and making people laugh—it fires me up. The thought of being on stage makes me so excited I could cry. And what if I could do that for a damn living?

What if I could travel and speak on stages? Holy shit, there it is—combining the two things I love in one package. And bring my nephew Malikai with me? *Sheeeeiiiit*, now we've got a to-do list.

Once I knew this idea was it, then I thought, *How the hell do I get there?*

The first problem was that I was making close to nothing at my job. I had gotten into some debt, I was fine, and everything was good—but I wasn't *moving* forward.

There's a place of complacency you do not want to stay in. I knew I needed to figure out my job situation, as making money being a speaker, coach, and author is the long game—like the *long* game—and I knew that would take years to become profitable.

I went back to Allie and told her about money woes. She said I should come and sell for her. I would make 100 percent commission, but I could make $10,000 per month, if not more. I heard 100 percent commission and shut the door. *Nope, that ain't me.*

You see, I had a block about sales because my dad has been grinding his entire career in the car business. I told Allie, and she said, "Look, this isn't the car business. You'd work from home and take calls, and I will teach you how to sell. If you go the business route, you'll need to learn this anyway, and you'll be around business owners."

I still said no—until a few months later, when I chose to move home because I hated paying my apartment complex money when all I could do was work to pay them. It was time for me to enter the world of sales.

My dad had told me forever that I was meant for it; I had the gift he had, communication skills. "You can talk to and relate to anyone," he said, "and that cannot be taught."

I'll never forget talking to my dad about this thing with Allie, and he knew Allie from years back. He knew how successful she was. He said, "You need to hitch your wagon to that redheaded chick and never look back."

And that's what I did.

Pivotal moment: I realized it's not what you know; it is *who* you *choose* to listen to. I listened to my dad, and I listened to Allie—a person who was where I wanted to be.

A spark was lit—I'll be damned.

In twelve months, I had managed to 10X my entire life. By living at home, I could spend more time with my nephew, who spends half his time there. I could pay my parents rent instead of some property company. I was able to send my parents on a first-class trip to Hawaii with all expenses paid. I started my own business, started writing a book, started a podcast (Darian told me to start one, and I listened). Now, I am working on building a coaching business, and as I write this, I've just been accepted to speak at an international women's conference.

All of this is in motion so that I can live the life I have always dreamt for myself. It's not about getting rich; it's about living my life authentically and doing what I love, helping people in a way I wasn't. It's about being able to retire my parents and teach my niece and nephew how to do the same for their own lives.

I have always noticed people like professional athletes or musicians—seeing the passion they have for what they do while they're playing performing. I envision myself on that stage. I've at least got to try.

You'll fail sometimes—I know I will—that's part of the game.

What's that Michael Jordan quote again? I'll tell you: "I've missed more than nine thousand shots in my career. I've lost almost three hundred games. Twenty-six times, I've been trusted to take the game-winning shot and missed." And that's Michael freakin' Jordan.

You know what being ballin' with a side of bipolar means?

It's going through your trauma, coming out of it, fighting for your life tooth and nail, and finding out who you want to be for the rest of your life—and then working toward that dream.

What is your "stage"? Go in that direction.

If it truly makes you so excited and nervous, and you have a good gut feeling, you've gotta go do it.

(*Note*: if it's not safe, happy, and healthy—or if you have a bad gut feeling, and it makes you nervous—probably don't do that thing.)

At least you can say you went toward your dreams. You'll figure out something along the way that will work for you.

Being in love with being alive means not having to depend on someone else for your own happiness. You should love your life in such a way that you don't need to find the partner of your dreams to make you happy.

If someone came up to me, and they were just as awesome as I was, and they said, "Let's try this," I'd say, "Sure, come *join me* in my amazing life. Let's share this shit."

If there is something in your life you want to change, change it.

If you want to look better, go do it.

If you want to feel better, eat better, or take better care of your body, go on a health journey.

If you want to make more money, then get a better job or learn the skill of sales—no one can take that skill away from you, and once you know how to sell something, you can sell anything, anywhere.

If you want to find a hobby, to start a business, or to write a book, do the damn thing.

Through this journey, you'll find out what you truly love—and what you don't too.

I thought I was going to be a real estate agent. I learned that wasn't for me.

It's okay to try things and learn they're not for you—it's the clarity we're looking for.

To work on your dream, you must gain three things:

- Clarity—understanding what your goal truly is.
- Commitment—having determination and focus to get to your goal.
- Tenacity—grasping ahold of and staying true to this goal no matter what happens.

First, you need clarity. Then you see the goal, and then you focus on and commit to it. But without the tenacity to never give up when life happens, you'll quit the first time a storm hits.

Once you ask yourself what lights your fire and what you want your Super Bowl to be, listen to the right people. Talk to people who are where you want to be. Listen to or read the right kinds of books that feed your soul for the good. Learn, do, and be.

Takeaways

If you made it to this book, that means you survived whatever trauma has happened in your life. Use that trauma for good. What did you learn? How much stronger are you now? What and who do you want to be for the rest of your life?

What lights your fire?

LET'S GO!

Chapter 14
You Only Have Control over What You Can Control

"I cannot always control what goes on outside.
But I can always control what goes on inside."
—Wayne Dyer

Let's talk about control—or lack thereof.

In AA, they say the Serenity Prayer: "God, grant me the serenity to accept the things I cannot change, the courage to change the things I can, and the wisdom to know the difference."

We cannot change other people. We can only control our reactions, effort, and attitude.

Now trust me: I have a big problem with understanding this principle, because there are times in life when things can get tough, especially if a challenge has to do with a child. It's very hard to understand that you can only control yourself and not others if a loved one is involved, so hear me when I say I totally understand the struggle.

But ultimately, worry, fear, and doubt are things we must let go of in our lives. What you focus on, you create more of.

When I talk about learning to be in love with being alive, all this means is taking responsibility for our lives. Part of that is taking control but also letting go.

There's no need for me to *need* anyone to like me. I know the important people love me and are there. If you don't have people like that in your life, you can go find them. I went to an Al-Anon meeting one time, and it was great. I want to go back, I just haven't. The people in that room heard a little bit about what I was worried about, and I had so much support from strangers—it was unreal. At least five people came up to me and gave me a hug after I'd shared for five minutes; those people could have become my entire support system, based on one meeting. If you don't have people, go find them—they are out there.

You also cannot let emotion take over your life when it comes to others affecting you and your mental well-being. Here's what my therapist told me after a rant and vent session about a fight my sister and I got into. She said, "You are letting her, and this fight rule your entire existence. You need to be a basketball of emotions. Right now, you have a bubble."

She meant when you have a little bubble around you, it can be popped at any time, by any asshole. But when you build a basketball around you? Shit, you become untouchable.

Once you have your bipolar world in order, you have your routine, and your values and personality are back, and on top of that, you are a basketball of emotion—no one can touch you.

Do not be a people pleaser. Say no when you want to say no. Do the thing when you want to do the thing. You can have control over yourself, how you react to life, and your disorder—not much else. And that's okay. Give it to God, the universe, or source energy and move on.

I'll tell you this about that (my dad says that all the time): you've gotta get used to getting rid of toxic people. My grandma and my dad always say, "Misery loves company." If someone is miserable, they will pour all that trash on you. It is not on you to solve the world's problems.

We can help people. We can share insight, experience, advice, and so on—but we cannot make people happy, nor can we make people change or live the way we want them to.

If someone treats you badly, or if you're in an abusive or toxic relationship, get rid of them.

Here's the true question. If you hang out with someone, ask yourself this: *Did I feel good about myself when I was around that person?* If not, get rid of them. Now, some people can fool you and suck you into their own mess, and that's just something you'll have to decipher. If people are mean to others, get rid of them.

I heard Oprah quote Maya Angelou, with advice that I love: "When people show you who they are, believe them."

Here's some Phylecia wisdom I'm gonna throw at you real quick. (A lot is from AA tenets, which I learned from my dad.)

Principles to live by:

- Do the next right thing. (I can't tell you how many times random things just work out, and I think it's the universe paying it forward or repaying me for doing the next right thing the month before. When you do the next right thing, the stars begin to align. It may not take a week, but you'll get there.)
- Keep your side of the road clean.
- Do good and be good.
- Don't lie, don't cheat, and don't steal.

- Be kind—to your neighbor, to the guy at the gas station, to the chick in the bathroom.
- Add value to whomever you talk to throughout the day.
- Stay humble.
- Throw good and love into the world; what goes around comes around.
- Be the support system you want to have in place in your own life.
- Help others.
- Live with a glass-half-full mindset.
- Drugs and alcohol do not help.
- Nothing lasts. Remember the good times on the bad days and know the bad days won't last forever.
- Say what you mean and mean what you say.
- If you have a chip on your shoulder, figure it out.
- Get clear on what you want out of life and go do it.
- If you want to be great at your job, or have a great career, find it.
- If you've always wanted to do something, and it's always on your mind, find a way to get it done.
- Figure out what makes you sad or self-conscious and try to get rid of it or fix it.
- Know yourself and what you need in each moment:
    - when to reflect, and when to rejoice
    - when to lie flat on the floor and breathe

  - when to ponder, and when to come up with your next plan.
  - when to move and have your own dance party
  - when to listen to a book or music
  - when to be productive vs. relaxing—not being lazy, although that's glorious when deserved.
- When you know you messed up, take responsibility, not feeling guilty but solving the problem.
- If you party, be smart, be responsible, and don't put yourself or others in danger.
- It's okay to have fun, but not reckless.
- Know when to be alone, or when you need your own space.
- Know when you need to be with friends or family.
- Know when you need to figure something out on your own, and when to ask for help.
- Know when to listen to advice and implement it.
- Know who to come to for certain things, and who not to come to for certain things, such as questions about money, life, your career, and the big picture.
- Know who to ask for the hard truth and who to go to when you need someone to be soft.
- Know that while bipolar is an explanation, it is not an excuse. That card cannot be played forever.
- See the beauty in life but understand the storms.
- Choose to see the light instead of always seeing the darkness.

- Rain and getting lost or stuck bring character to the day—as long as you have a plan, and you are safe and prepared.
- If it's safe, happy, and healthy, rock on.
- If you feel good about something in your gut—if it excites you but makes you nervous—you gotta do it.
- Know when something doesn't feel right in your gut. Be in tune with your star player (Katt Williams's expression): if it doesn't feel right, don't do it, or get out of it.
- Get rid of assholes in your life; you don't need 'em.
- Try new things to find out what you love and what you hate.
- Know when to push through anxiety and get comfortable being uncomfortable. Also know when anxiety or discomfort is unnecessary, and you can get rid of it.

Core values when it comes to living with and being bipolar:

- Whenever something happens, you begin to flail, or shit's going awry, *go back to basics*: Stage 3, then Stage 4.
- You must come into every day prepared and intentional. Fight for your life every single day until it becomes second nature. You are going to become stronger than this dumb-ass disorder ever was. This thing does not win.

- As you begin to take control, you'll get more advanced. It will still be the same cycle, but instead of survival, you'll begin to help others. You'll begin to grow.
- Do not fuck with a victim mentality—that's for suckers. When we're ballin', we take responsibility for our lives. We all know it's not fair, but if you live on that pity pot, you'll be a sad sack forever. And no one wants to be a sad sack. Remember, no one is coming to save you. You must save yourself. This is your fight, no one else's.
- In the beginning, stability is your number one job. It stays your number one job for life, but it begins to get easier and feel more normal.
- Have a plan for mania and a plan to get out of depression. We don't feed the black wolf that is depressed, but also, when we're bipolar, feeding the white wolf too much can make it turn to gold—and then we fly to the sun. We must stay centered.
- You're going to get your disorder down to a science.
- Know the answers to these questions:
    - What calms you down and relaxes you?
    - What do you enjoy? How can you laugh every day?
    - What brings you confidence? Independence? Joy? Self-worth? (The saddest people I've ever known struggle because they don't have self-worth, confidence, and independence. If you have those

things, how could you not be striving to live your best life? You must know *what* will bring you those qualities; then, figure out *how* to get there.)
    - What excites you?
- Don't let fear stop you; just have a plan.
- Reflect on your journey, where you've been, and how far you've come.
- When you feel stuck in the day-to-day, do one thing that will make you laugh or feel productive.
- You must have total belief and determination.
- Find gratitude every day.

If you live by these foundational rules, I promise happiness follows. You'll find out what you love to do just by doing these things. Your own positivity and kindness will reveal what you love and who you want to be.

Takeaways

Maya Angelou said, "I've learned that people will forget what you said, people will forget what you did, but people will never forget how you made them feel." I love making people feel good about themselves because they repay it by showing kindness, whether to me or to others. Conducting ourselves in this way truly makes the world a better place to be.

Chapter 15
Finding Purpose in Each Season of Your Life

"The meaning of life is to find your gift. The purpose of life is to give it away."

—Pablo Picasso

If life is going to happen no matter what, why don't we try to find joy in every single day? Find gratitude on the shitty days and make them just a little bit brighter. What value can you find each day? How can you make a not-so-good experience meaningful?

I think purpose is often misunderstood. We have been taught as a society that we all have one purpose, and it is our duty as humans to find it.

That puts a lot of pressure on us.

In some seasons of your life, your purpose is getting stable. In other seasons, it may be to raise kids. Your purpose might be going on a health journey and getting fit. Sometimes your purpose is mundane as hell—just survival. You choose your purpose, and it changes in different phases of your life.

When I was sixteen years old and Mormon, I was given what's called a "patriarchal blessing." It's a blessing that tells you what your path in life will look like. Mine said things like "Phylecia, you're a daughter of Heavenly Father" (which is fine) and "You will marry a man and be an incredible mother."

So my whole young life, I thought, *Okay, that's my path. I'll be a wife and mother.* If people who know me personally read that, they'd laugh. Because that is not me. Like at all (at least not right now).

My motivations are different from yours. My purpose is different from yours. You choose what you want your purpose to be, and you go do it.

Just know it changes when life changes. Sometimes, we're just hoping we go to work without losing our shit. That's fine—that's still the purpose.

Are you with me?

There was a time in my life when my purpose was getting my life and personality back.

Then my nephew was born, and it was no longer about me. My purpose was him. He was and is the center of my universe.

Now, my family has nailed how we are going to raise these kids, and it's time for me to focus on my own dreams. But a dream without a goal and a to-do list will stay a dream forever.

When your purpose is getting stable, you also don't abandon your responsibilities. If you have kids or people who depend on you, you still put stability and getting level as your number one priority. You take care of them too, but if you do not put your mental health first, your kids or family will suffer in the long term.

Remember, when we're talking about purpose, it's not all about you all the time. There will come times when it's your turn to add value to other people's lives.

Takeaways

Don't put so much pressure on finding your "one true purpose." It will change throughout your life, and guess what? You can design your own purpose for each season of this path we're on.

Chapter 16
Staying Centered

"Tomorrow is a new day. It has never been touched."

—Modern Love

The last chapter—can you believe it?

Staying centered in your life needs to become your long-term focus. It is our duty to take responsibility and ownership of our lives. Over the course of your own Bipolar Life Cycle, you will begin to thrive just as I've described in this book. But that does not mean you can get cocky.

We need to respect this disorder. We cannot forget that it is a matter of *when*, not if, we will fall or fly too high.

Staying centered every single day is of utmost importance. I do daily check-ins. While I work out, I say my affirmations, prayers, and mantras. I make sure I am centered and feel at peace. If I feel centered and at peace, that's a good sign, and I'll go on about my day.

But as you know with bipolar, things can take a quick turn at any time of the day. That's when we go back to basics and our cycle so that we can interrupt the loop of depression or ensure we won't fly to the sun in mania.

For me, staying centered also means staying organized. I don't want to live in anarchy. Being clean and keeping your home or living space clean are important for your mental health.

When I lived in my apartment, each time I entered, I would take a breath of air, exhale, and love being in my home. It was peaceful and clean. That's how you want to feel internally too.

Organize your life, get a calendar, and make lists. Block out time for relaxation, for fun, for productivity. There are always spaces in time that you can work on yourself. I have my days scheduled down to the minute.

What I find works is dividing my life into three categories, as having three things to focus on doesn't overwhelm me. Then I have achievable action steps for each category each week, and I make these my mantras daily.

For example:

Category 1: mental stability and physical health

Subcategories: daily meds, supplements, diet, exercise

Category 2: professional life (my job and business)

Subcategories: focusing on sales training every day, thinking about what I can do daily to move the needle for my business, podcast, book, and other content

Category 3: nephew, family, friends

Subcategories: ensuring my nephew has everything he needs and gets taken to sports, spending quality time with him and my niece, figuring out what my parents and friends need, being present

Your categories are going to be different depending on where you are, and these will change over time, but I find focusing on three areas and then having baby steps for each one makes things easier to attain. Rather than trying to keep twenty thoughts in your mind, write things down, focus, and keep it simple.

Don't forget that if you do get overwhelmed and crash, bipolar will sink in. It's like a devil. When it sees a weakness, it creeps in. That's why daily check-ins are paramount.

Now, when you notice yourself slipping, you have tools. Go back to Stage 3 of the Bipolar Life Cycle mentioned in Part I: routine, medications, solutions, and a plan of attack. Start each day prepared to fight back.

When things get easy, or when you begin searching, ask yourself: *What am I searching for? What do I enjoy? What do I love? Who do I want to be?*

If bipolar sinks in, relax. Identify it, and work on your solutions.

If bipolar success were divided into four boxes, this is what each would contain (find the diagram at ballinandbipolar.com/free-resources):

Box 1—Stability. This means getting level on medications, finding the right doctors and support system, and understanding your own diagnosis, your triggers, your onsets. It includes finding your solutions to mania and depression, being prepared and intentional each day to fight back, and keeping up with your daily routine, check-ins, mantras, sleep, healthy eating, and exercise.

Box 2—Gratitude and Mindset. If you go into every day with gratitude, the right mindset will follow. Belief system is here too.

Box 3—CIJ (Confidence, Independence, and Joy). The sources of these feelings will change over time, and you'll become more advanced in your growth over time. But focus on these three things every day.

Box 4—Asking the Right Questions. Ask yourself: *How can I be better? How can I live better in this experience? Who can I help?*

If you are constantly working on these four areas, the simple math of it is progression and momentum. We will all struggle sometimes, but if you keep these four categories in mind every day, you will see the light in your days. You will become stronger, and you will find your own success and path forward.

I want to talk to you about something I am just now learning about. It's the Law of Attraction. I have to mention Rachel Hollis one more time (if you don't know by now, she is my idol). It was an episode of her podcast, which everyone should listen to; it's amazing. She was interviewing spiritual teacher Michael Beckwith, and I was all in. They were speaking about the idea that positive people attract positivity, while negative people attract negativity.

Some of the things they said resonated with me 100 percent.

According to Verywell Mind, the Law of Attraction states:

the energy of your thoughts manifests your experiences. So positive thoughts manifest positive experiences and vice versa. Advocates suggest there are central universal principles that make up the law of attraction [including]:

> **Like attracts like**: This law suggests that similar things are attracted to one another. It means that people tend to attract people who are similar to them—but it also suggests that people's thoughts tend to attract similar results. Negative thinking is believed to attract negative experiences, while positive thinking is believed to produce desirable experiences.

This idea could be controversial, but I did a podcast episode about this if you'd like to listen. Believing you are depressed or debilitated and cannot live a normal life means you *will never* live a normal life, because that is your mindset. On the flip side, if you believe in and are determined and intentional about getting better, you will get better. You must be intentional about it every single day, though.

First, you must come to believe that depression can leave. If it can leave, that means we can find the solution to get out of it. I have been there. I fought and fought until it became a math problem. I know exactly what I'm going to do when depression hits, and as I fight harder every day, coming into everyday life with the intention to be light and happy, the clouds disappear for longer amounts of time. That's where you will get. At some point, the clouds may go away for years, but you will know what to do when the next storm hits.

If you believe that you are going to find joy today, you will consciously look for the joy in your day. If you believe that you are miserable, you will stay miserable. Remember, you cannot think your way out of depression, distracting your brain long enough that the focus isn't on how shitty you feel. The focus is physically elsewhere.

Ask the right questions: *How can I get out of this?* If I did, so can you.

Here are some ideas I want to leave you with.

Ask yourself, *How can I make my current situation better?* This means you are looking toward the solution.

Sometimes I think that unfortunately, people are okay being miserable. You can get comfortable being sad. It's tempting to continue to be sad and complain about how you're bipolar and your life sucks.

You know what's hard as shit? Telling yourself you're going to get up, you're going to find the damn beauty in the day, and you're going to help

> someone else because that's the only way you will feel better. That shit is hard to do.
>
> It's hard being depressed, and it's hard to fight back. But if you do fight, your life can be beautiful.

One more tiny thought to leave you with: I want to talk about football again. Why football, you ask?

Because we do not compare our first quarter with someone else's fourth, or vice versa. If you are playing peewee football, you don't even know how to play the damn game yet—so don't compare yourself to Tom Brady! That makes no sense.

This is *your* game. You learn the rules of the game and how to play, and then you enter that field prepared to deal with the bipolar flags on the play that will come.

The flags on the play are inevitable, but if you know the rules, you may gain some yardage. Or you may lose some. You may be able to kick a field goal. Who knows? When bipolar tackles you, get right back up. The ball is yours. Get to the next down and keep trucking.

If you're in your fourth quarter, go help someone who's only in their first. Show them the ropes.

Now, at the very least, I hope that you have hope and guidance for this thing called bipolar. I have walked in your shoes. I have felt like my entire life was a lie and there was no coming back. I mourned the loss of myself and my past life.

Make this book your own, and let's go to work.

This is your life and your fight—and you are worth every single second.

Now, go be happy or get the F* out.

With all the love and support in the world,

Phylecia

Here's What to Do Next

Whenever you're ready, here are four ways I'd like to help you take the next step on your journey:

1. Access All Your Free Bonuses

By reading this book and saying yes to yourself, you have unlocked every bonus and resource in this book.

Visit **ballinandbipolar.com/free-resources** to get all the freebies!

You come up with your own solutions, confidence, independence, and joy and whatever they mean to you.

Fill out your own Bipolar Life Cycle so that you have a true game plan and the yellow brick road I never had. That's the way out of this thing.

2. Join Me in Becoming Ballin' and Bipolar

If you'd like to chat about how my team and I may be able to help you on your journey, I invite you to visit **ballinandbipolar.com** to schedule a call to discuss your bipolar success plan.

3. Hire Phylecia to Speak!

If you are looking for a high-energy hype man of a motivational speaker for your conference, event, or mastermind, I'd love to bring it!

Email **phylecia@ballinandbipolar.com** with "SPEAKING" in the subject line.

4. Connect on Social Media

Let's keep the convo going! The journey doesn't end here. I'd love to connect with you on all social platforms. Let's have some fun!

You can find me on socials at:

Instagram: @phylecia_ballinandbipolar01

Podcast: Ballin and Bipolar (all outlets)

Facebook: Phylecia - Ballin & Bipolar - Bipolar Success Coaching

Facebook Group: Ballin & Bipolar - Our Support Space!!

Website: ballinandbipolar.com

Acknowledgments

My mom and dad, Jeana and Raymond—for catching me when I fell

Darian—for being my forever cheerleader

Amanda and Jon—for getting me help when I needed it most

Ashley—for being there no matter the circumstances and having these beautiful kids of yours

Malikai—for helping me learn what true love really is; you are my pure joy, sweet boy

Brielle—for bringing even more joy and sunshine to our lives

Allie—for giving me the ultimate clarity I needed and being the best mentor, boss, and friend

Carolyn and Katie—for never wavering

Krystina and Nick—for being my comfort in the hardest days

Noelle, Ian, and Shane—for being the support I needed in the worst part of my life

Riley and Smokey—for bringing me back to life

Pam—for teaching me to keep trudging forward

Dr. Ron—for getting me level and diagnosing the right disorder

BIB team (especially Adrienne Dyer!)—for helping me write this damn thing!

All the people in my corner—you know who you are

About the Author

Written by Allie Bloyd
Friend, mentor, and lifelong cheerleader

When I was eighteen years old, I returned home for the summer after my freshman year of college and was looking for a summer job. I had heard from a girl at school that she had served at Cracker Barrel for a few years and did pretty well, so I decided to apply. That's when I met Phylecia.

I was instantly drawn to her energy and enthusiasm. She always had a smile on her face, and we very quickly hit it off. Everyone loved her. We were always laughing, singing, and dancing in the kitchen, spending our lunch break in my car while pulling twelve-hour double shifts. We talked about everything under the sun and felt a unique connection from the beginning.

We had some mutual friends and began to hang out outside of work, seeing each other more regularly as the months went by. Then, something changed.

We had all gathered at Phylecia's apartment one night to hang out, and something was off. We all felt it. She was talking a mile a minute, and while that wasn't completely abnormal for her, this was different. She was not acting like herself, and we all left early, confused and concerned.

I decided to go back to her apartment the next day to check on her, and when I did, I only grew more worried. I learned the next day that she was admitted to a psychiatric facility, and shortly after, I found out that she was diagnosed with bipolar disorder and what we had witnessed was full-blown mania.

It was a very hard time for me and everyone who knew and loved her. After she was released, we weren't sure what to expect. Would this be the same girl that we knew and loved, or would she be different? Would she still wanna hang out with us? Would she remember anything that happened? We didn't know, but we did know that we wanted to be there for her.

We still hung out, and I did my best to support her, but things were different for a while. After I left Cracker Barrel, we saw each other less but continued to stay in touch over the years.

I got married and started a family and still considered her to be one of my closest friends, though we saw much less of each other. Then, a few years down the road, we had plans to hang out one night, but she backed out. She felt like I was doing so much more with my life than she was, and it made her feel bad about herself. I was incredibly hurt and saddened, but I understood. I prayed for so long that she would see herself as the person I saw her to be: someone smart, beautiful, and strong—an overcomer.

After that, we fell out of touch for a while, until one day, she reached out. I had started a business, and it was doing well, and she wanted advice about work, finances, and life in general. We continued to talk, and she shared her hopes and dreams, which I fully encouraged her to pursue.

One day when we were talking about her job, how unfulfilled she felt at work, and how she wanted to make more money, I told her that I thought she would be a perfect fit for sales, despite her longtime resistance to the field.

I was in a position where I needed to hire a new closer for my sales team and told her that if she was willing to go in on this and give it a try, I knew it could change her life. It would give her the ability to look behind the scenes of the thriving coaching business, to get coaching from me on her business aspirations, and to hone the ability to find fulfillment and financial stability in her work for the first time.

It was a big leap of faith for her to leave her job and come on board, but she did it with the desire to learn, grow, and thrive. And that's exactly what she did. Over the next year, she dedicated herself to learning the art of sales and pursuing her business dreams. It completely changed her life.

I've seen her grow personally and professionally in such incredible ways over the last several years. Now, I am so thankful to see her fulfill this lifelong dream of writing a book, sharing her unique voice and experiences to give hope to others. I know that she will change the lives of others with bipolar disorder and beyond, in the same way that she has changed her own.

You're in for a wild ride!

Made in the USA
Middletown, DE
03 March 2025

72134981R00134